MIND
PROGRAMMING
TECHNIQUES

Shape Your Destiny, Reprogram Your
Subconscious Through Psychological Techniques
And Thoughts Control, Develop Willpower And
Habits To Achieve Success

ARIANNA PETERSON

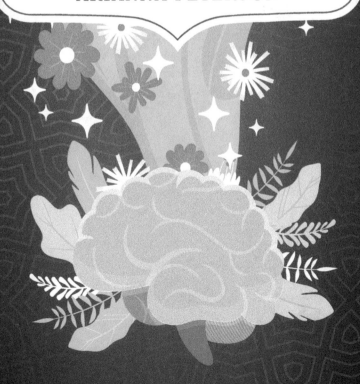

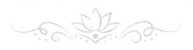

Introduction

Famous philosophers and scientists have for hundreds of years been investigating the human mind, or as some would call it, the brain. This organ is more than just the central processor of our bodies. Theories of how our brains work have developed, been disproven, revived, and then recanted again. As science progresses, we can verify certain premises of research, which were previously only unproven theories. We are, for instance, able to see into the brain, track where memories form and even measure the electrical impulses that carry thought by using advanced imaging equipment. In a sense, we can now "see" our thoughts. This is not unlike the movie *Johnny Mnemonic*, in which the brain is visualized as a storage mechanism that can be used to retain specific information. However, in the past, we believed that we were unable to control what the brain remembered, or how it remembered. Recently, we have discovered that, like in the movie, where Keanu Reeves' character ditches his childhood memories, we can also take control of our memories. We can select which memories will affect us and how. Through advanced programming techniques, we can even "erase" the impact of negative memories. Hence, if you had a traumatic childhood, you can be the director of your brain's movie and edit those scenes that have been determining how you see life.

René Descartes, renowned 17th-century mathematician and an important scientific mind of his era, famously theorized that it was not about having an excellent mental capacity (or our minds) but rather about how well we use that mind. This notion highlights two aspects of mindful living: that we need to develop a good mind, and that we must be able to use it. If we are to believe this reasoning, then we are able to become the creators of our life. In developing a good mind and learning how to use it, we can determine where we end up and what we achieve. We can become the captain of our life's boat. However, this will only happen when we start forming new thinking patterns that will fill your sails and not continue to sink your boat.

The human brain is an awesomely powerful mechanism. It controls how we think, what we think, and how we feel about that thought. We have only recently begun to formulate theories that explore how to change our mindset by using our mind and science to create a new life outlook and decision-making paradigm.

The Theory

Before you can begin to program your mind to achieve your greatest wishes, some concepts need to be explained. It is not a magic trick, and you can't simply make it so by wishing for it. Truly, "if wishes were horses, beggars would ride." You need to understand how your operational systems are wired into your brain and the effects these have on your thinking before you can redesign your thinking and move forward. It's not as simple as choosing between Windows and Mac. The process takes time, and there will be some really amazing leaps forward as well as the occasional setback. However, with concerted efforts and a firm grasp on the theory that underpins these dramatic changes that you are about to embark on (and a pinch of determination), you will be able to change your mind and harness its power to free you from leading a life that may not feel worth living. Happily, there have been some giants who walked before you, and now it's simply a matter of following in their tracks. The path is laid before you – just take the first step.

The Tool

Once you understand how the mind works, you will begin a spectacular journey that will take you to places you had never imagined in your life while also leading you closer to your authentic life. Fortunately, there are some tools that you can pack in your bag that you take on this journey. You will learn how to use imagination, autosuggestion, and visualization, combined with powerful meditations, to build your internal communication skills. This will allow you to run your life like a ship where the crew all know their places, they are devoted to their captain, and they do all that they can to reach their destination.

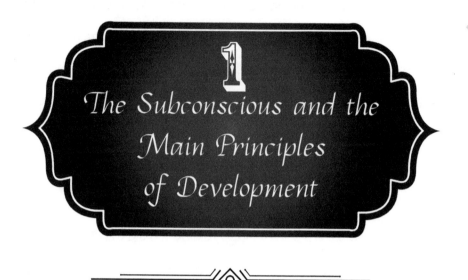

1

The Subconscious and the Main Principles of Development

The human brain is a truly magnificent organ. It controls how we think, what we believe, how we feel about those thoughts, and even determines our actions upon those thoughts. The estimated 100 billion neural cells (WebMD.com, n.d.) create an intricate network that processes, makes, responds to, and stores our thoughts. The brain is the tangible aspect of the much more intangible concept, namely the mind.

The two words are often used as being mutually inclusive, yet, in reality, they tend to be more mutually exclusive. The brain may contain the mind, but where exactly it sits within those 100 billion neural cells is still the topic of ongoing research. However, psychologists have developed their theories over the years. Even in historic times, the Ancient Greeks had already theorized about where the mind sits. For lack of a better word at that time, they referred to this as the soul seat, and if the human soul did have a seat, that seat would be in mind, not the brain.

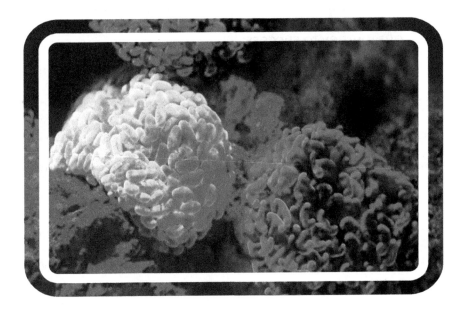

(Image 1.1)

The subconscious mind is the one that pulls our strings, and though we may believe that we are in control of our conscious mind, we are, in fact, entirely at the mercy of our instincts, drives, and experiences that are stored and created in the subconscious mind. (Image 1.2)

The notion of the mind also having parts, like the brain has physical hemispheres, was first formalized by Sigmund Freud in 1915 when he theorized that reason consists of a conscious, preconscious, and subconscious part. He continued to explore how the mind can be stimulated to change our perceptions of our experiences. Now, more than a hundred years later, we are continuing that research and finding ways to use the power of this knowledge to drive our journey to success.

The successful development of our minds and the application of those minds in our daily lives is about successfully changing our perceptions. In essence, our perceptions are how we understand, interpret, and react to something. Writer and philosopher Aldus Huxley famously wrote, "Here are things known, and there are things unknown, and in between are the doors of perception." We can only change our perceptions - we cannot change events. Therefore, we can only change our perceptions. To do that successfully and lead better and more fulfilling lives, we need to explore, understand, and change the world of our subconscious mind.

What Is the Subconscious?

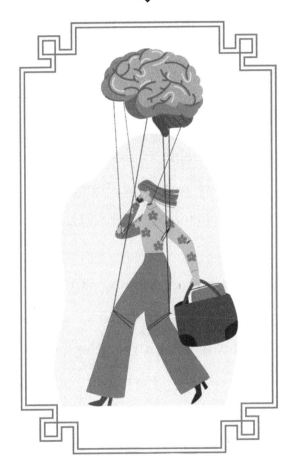

(Image 1.2)

The subconscious mind is the one that pulls our strings, and though we may believe that we are in control of our conscious mind, we are, in fact, quite at the mercy of our instincts, drives, and experiences that are stored and created in the subconscious mind. (Image 1.2)

Stop. Take a deep breath. Did you think about that breath? You undoubtedly did - since you were told to. However, do you have to think about every breath you take? No. This and other reactions such as digestion, heartbeat, blood circulation, and a gazillion other intricate systems that keep our bodies running are all controlled by what scientists call the autonomic nervous system. It's our body's co-pilot that helps to run things while we, the captain, are elsewhere occupied. These jumpy autonomic system activities are, in turn, governed by the subconscious mind.

Bruce Lipton, a famous scientist and also an author of several ground-breaking books, posits that the subconscious mind is a tape recorder or CD writer that stores every experience we have ever had and plays back the highlights (as habits) to direct our lives. We are, of course, not able to physically see the subconscious mind. Scientists have not yet identified the particular collection of cells in our body that forms the subconscious mind. Perhaps with continued research, we may one day be able to pinpoint precisely where the subconscious lies. However, we have been able to discover a few scientifically proven facts about the subconscious mind. For instance, it operates independently from the conscious mind, and there is very little measurable interaction between the conscious and subconscious mind. Hence, we can't switch off the tape that plays non-stop throughout our lives. It's like a dance instructor that yells to us what steps to make and rhythm to follow, which we follow without question, effectively rendering us as marionettes with the subconscious holding the strings.

If that image leaves you feeling quite depressed, don't despair. We have also discovered ways to communicate with the subconscious mind and take back control, but we can't simply "talk" to it. Ziogas[1] (2018) reasons that it is vitally important to gain control over our subconscious mind as it controls our lives and experiences. This means that if we wish to achieve our deepest wishes and live with a purpose to reach our desired goals, then we need to master the power of our subconscious mind.

Brian Tracy (n.d.), an international life coach and public speaker, defines the subconscious as "like a huge memory

---

[1]Ziogas, G.J. (2018). How To Reprogram Your Subconscious Mind: A Step-By-Step Guide. www.medium.com

bank. Its capacity is virtually unlimited, and it permanently stores everything that ever happens to you." He does not mention here that we are completely unaware of the thoughts, experiences, and emotions stored in our subconscious mind. These thoughts, experiences, and emotions become the habits that we follow in life. We are, in a sense, preprogrammed to behave in a certain way. For example, if you had a bad experience in a swimming pool as a child, the memory will have stuck in your subconscious mind. Later in life, you may still not like swimming and may even prefer showering instead of bathing (which involves immersion in water, similar to being in a swimming pool). The subconscious mind's directions determine this habit of thinking or feeling. It issues these directions through emotional responses to situations we face in our daily lives. What can be detrimental to our progress through life is that we are completely unaware of our habits or biases that the subconscious mind imposes on us. This means that the subconscious mind is the pilot of your life, instead of that responsibility and power resting in your hands.

According to research, the subconscious mind is initially a blank slate at birth. It bar a few instinctual drives, such as the survival and procreation drives (Kendra, 2019) that are concerned with preserving life and propagation. Freud, who gave us the field of psychoanalysis and defined the mind's structure, believed that the subconscious mind is programmed with our experiences. All of them! These experiences, events, and our emotional reactions to these events (whether we consciously perceive them or not) are what begin to write on the blank slate that we are at birth. The subconscious mind, which, up until then, had been merely concerned with maintaining the physical homeostasis or balance of our physical processes such as breathing and digestion, then also takes on the mantle of maintaining our congruence or stability as mental and physical beings. Tracy (n.d.) finds that our subconscious minds maintain our homeostasis and mental stability. It ensures that there is congruence between our actions and our words. This means that the subconscious mind is responsible for determining how our bodies function, but it also determines how our minds and perceptions work. Our past then begins to predict our future.

The Subconscious and the Conscious Interaction

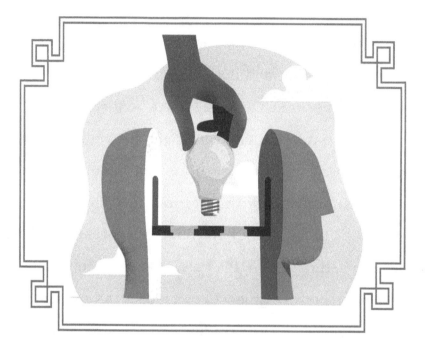

Lipton[2] (2019) remarks in his video speeches on YouTube that the subconscious mind is like a tape recorder and only stores information. The information is then transformed into the preprogrammed responses that your conscious mind follows. Therefore, the communication between the subconscious and the conscious mind will be

---

[2]Lipton, B. (2019). "I Can Teach You How to Program The Subconscious Mind"

a complicated matter. The subconscious mind is not a portion of the mind that reacts to or creates changes in our lives. We may think about change, but merely thinking it will not be enough to begin to change the programming that is already wired into our subconscious through a life-time of information.

So, how do the subconscious and conscious minds interact? If we can't simply talk to our subconscious, how do we control it? Mayer (2018) believes that we have better luck communicating with the subconscious mind through our emotions since that is how the subconscious mind communicates with us. Further, Mayer also points out that the subconscious mind, since it reacts more vital to a crisis (remember, its first encoded program is the life-instinct or survival program), will respond and interpret our instructions better with strong emotions. Unfortunately, the subconscious mind reacts strongly to threatening emotions such as fear or anxiety. It immediately initiates preprogrammed behavior to ensure our survival, such as becoming aggressive in new work environments or dominating our social partners to become the alpha of our pack.

From this discussion, it becomes clear that the communication is a bit one-sided. We can try and influence the subconscious mind through our emotions, but it can control how we act and our reactions to events and people. That's a bit like having a foreign taxi driver who rushes about and doesn't listen to a word you're trying to say, and the driver certainly doesn't listen to where you want to go. The problem is that we are thinking our instructions in words, while the subconscious mind since it began forming in our early childhood, has developed its language of communication. There might be some words that our subconscious mind can comprehend, but it is mostly the associations that are formed with words that it reacts to. Our subconscious mind does not hear the word "ball" and think logically about the word. The conscious mind might listen to the word "ball" and immediately form a mental picture of what the ball looks like and create a definition of the concept "ball" as being "a round object that is used in sports and child's play." However, the subconscious mind would instead respond with the feelings that the idea of "ball" brings. It can see the ball from our memories of having played with a ball. It can also experience the

15

feelings we had from our previous experiences with a ball, such as feeling happy as we played with a ball. The subconscious mind would then have a positive reaction to the idea of "ball" if it had previous favorable experiences involving a ball. It's like playing *Pictionary* with your taxi driver.

The subconscious mind is then able to respond better to emotionally laden images that convey new meanings. Through repetitive exposure to that emotion or image, it makes connections to habitualized thoughts and patterns. This is one of the reasons why music, sounds, smells, and visualizations are perhaps the most effective way to communicate with our subconscious minds. It may sound taxing to have to share using these ways, but it is how the subconscious mind first obtained the information that informed its decision-making habits and methods – through the senses (Papalia et al., 2008, p. 186-187)[3].

So, communication is possible from our end (the conscious mind), and the subconscious mind certainly knows how to send information our way. In the above

3 Papalia, D.E., Olds, S.W. & Feldman, R.D. (2008). *A Child's World: Infancy Through Adolescence* (11th ed.). McGraw-Hill: Boston.

paragraphs, the subconscious mind has sent several memories and associated feelings your way as you read. It may have sent you an image that you remembered of a foreign taxi driver when it encountered the word, and it made a connection to the idea of *Pictionary*. However, the subconscious mind can only respond to these if it relates to information that it already has in its vast memory stores. For instance, for someone who has never heard of *Pictionary*, this word would have no reaction other than confusion. The subconscious mind, therefore, retrieves information based on the stimulus we send it. Still, it does not change according to our wishes unless we can create entirely new memories and experiences to rewire our subconscious with new information.

The Structure of the Subconscious

We've already said that the subconscious mind is like a giant storehouse, a place where every experience or memory we've ever had is recorded. It is not unlike a portable or external hard drive for a computer. No matter how old the information on it becomes, it can always be retrieved again. The more recent the information, the easier it is to retrieve it, and the further back in our memories, something goes, the longer it may take to retrieve it.

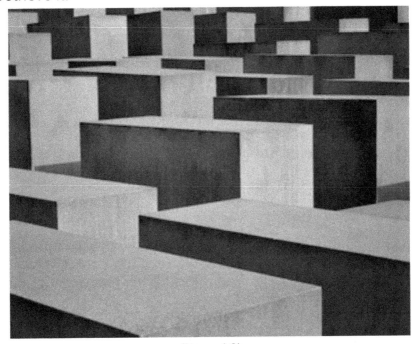

(Image 1.3)

The subconscious mind is a vast storeroom for all of our experiences and memories. (Image 1.3)

Understanding how the subconscious mind is structured can help us understand how it retrieves

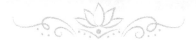

information based on new stimuli or events. This retrieved information is responsible for our decision-making process and emotions. We can think of the subconscious mind's structure as working as the operating system on your computer. If you are running on Windows 2000, you will not be able to do some of the things you can do with Windows 2010 or upwards. The main difference is that the system has been changed from the earlier version, allowing for new insights and connections to be made. Your subconscious mind is still stuck running on an outdated system, and as further information is received, the subconscious mind struggles to store it effectively. It ends up creating redundancy folders and chunking everything together as being "My Documents." Hence, it is unsurprising that our subconscious mind is structured so that all of the extra files can't flood back to the conscious mind. This is a necessary measure to ensure our system doesn't crash. Here's how it works (if you're wondering how the subconscious mind is structured concerning the whole mind

Sigmund Freud formulated a theory that our mind can be divided into three distinct sections. He termed this the "iceberg theory," and it works like this:

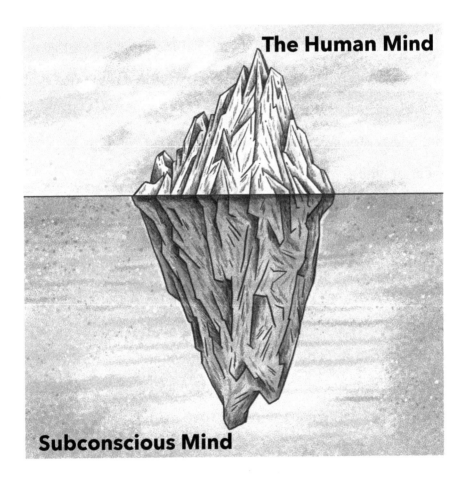

An iceberg (Image 1.4)

The human mind, like an iceberg, has visible parts, and that is our conscious mind. It has elements below the water, which are not as easily accessible, namely the subconscious mind. We can control the conscious mind. It is the logical center, where we are aware of our actions, and we can rationalize our decision making every day. Lipton (2019) believes that this part of our mind uses logic and creativity to overcome the challenges that do not fill us with fear (or challenges lacking an emotional response that would trigger the subconscious mind). Therefore, we can make decisions with this part of our mind, such as what to wear or where to park our car.

Below the line of consciousness (the waterline) is a much larger area of the mind, namely, the subconscious mind. It's also quite appropriate that the subconscious is compared to an iceberg, and the fact is that the area beneath the water is much larger and much more dangerous than what lies above the water. Suppose we are not able to recognize and create a positive relationship with our subconscious mind. In that case, it will wreck our lives just like the *Titanic* was sunk by an iceberg (specifically, its hidden parts under the water).

In between the tip of the iceberg and the parts hidden in the murky depths of our minds, we find a smaller section that is barely visible. This is called the preconscious mind, and it works like a type of filter to stop our subconscious mind from dredging up memories that are too traumatic to be conceptualized into our active thoughts. This filter keeps thoughts such as memories about traumatic events like child abuse, rape, and physical trauma hidden away to protect the conscious mind. However, this mechanism is placed under constant pressure as the subconscious mind can be triggered into releasing memories by conscious events or even emotions. Perhaps, for our purposes, the iceberg model can be substituted for the idea that the mind works like a funnel instead.

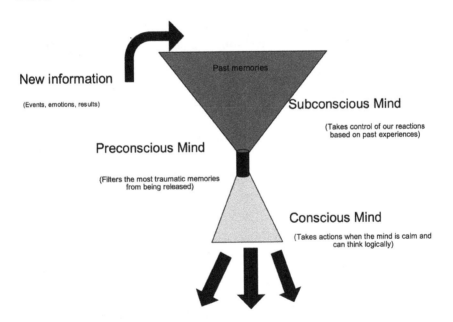

The mind as a funnel. (Figure 1.1)

In the above diagrammatic model, the subconscious acts like a sponge and it records non-stop, taking in new information into the brain. But, as anyone who's ever studied for a test, only to hit a blank wall when answering questions, will know, it is not so easy to retrieve information that we have studied. At times, it seems as if our whole world goes into the subconscious, but it doesn't come out into our conscious mind at the other end at all. It may be easy to state that our memories are all blocked because they are traumatic by the preconscious mind. And certainly, students would all agree that studying can be a traumatic business! However, it is not as simple as that.

The subconscious mind has to take the intangible and make it tangible so that it can be stored. Though the subconscious mind is a construct that we have created with psychological theories, it is still rooted in the physical world, namely our brain.

Information is coded into the brain via a complex network of neurons that form the brain matter. Through electrical impulses and chemical reactions, we retain the information, which is taken in by our senses. We see objects, people, and places while we hear sounds, language, and voices. These quantifiable bits of information are retained in the cells of the brain, where it can be accessed by the unconscious mind. If information is retrieved regularly, such as the easiest way to reach home from work, it becomes a habit. Quite literally, the neural pathways are strengthened to make that information easily found. Like a Google search, it pops up as the most searched information to your mind.

This is all great for daily routines that we don't necessarily want to focus on, such as getting dressed, making coffee, and knowing how to drive your car. But, unfortunately, we also form habits that are less useful, such as negative thinking habits like believing that we are not good enough, not loved, or that we will always be unhappy. If something has been drilled into us by a person in power during our childhood, such as a teacher, parent, or sports coach (Lipton, 2019), we will begin to form a neural pathway that makes that idea pop up on our subconscious mind's Google search every time. Whenever you think something (with your conscious mind) along the lines of "I am...," your wiring (in the subconscious mind) will lead to those habits that are so entrenched they have almost become highways and then complete the sentence for you. It might finish the sentence with "...not worthy" or "...not loveable." Old mental habits will then determine our thinking as a result.

Therefore, the physical structure of the mind with its neural wiring, its habit-forming encoding techniques, and the preprogrammed approach that thinks the first "search result" is the correct answer, is a powerful force in our lives. According to both Lipton (2019) and Tracy (n.d.)[4], we use the subconscious mind about 95% of the day, while the conscious mind is only operating 5% of the time. This means that we are directed and driven along by emotion-driven reactions, instead of consciously decided actions. The subconscious mind seeks to maintain a balance to sustain our biological processes, such as controlling breathing and metabolism, as well as maintaining our

---

[4]Tracy, B. (n.d.). Subconscious Mind Power Explained. Retrieved www.briantracy.com

mental stability by hiding traumatic events from our recall. Yet, it still trips us up in its quest for efficiency. Damaging beliefs can form when the subconscious has created information highways in our brain that links to negative memories or recorded memories that lead to building a negative mindset.

Subconscious Levels

Science has been able to effectively identify the different levels at which the human mind processes information. These levels are, in effect, frequencies that the different parts of the mind are most effective or suggestible at. By creating an electroencephalograph or brain graph (EEG), we can measure the frequency at which we think, according to Muse™ (2018). When we measure the brain's activities at the different stages of consciousness, we begin to understand some very interesting things.

Firstly, there is a frequency for each of our different states of consciousness. Sleep (which is our lowest state of consciousness) has a vibration or frequency called delta. This is the lowest frequency with the fewest vibrations. The brain is then in a state of rest, just like the sleep mode on your computer. By contrast, when we are busy writing tests or doing other mentally taxing tasks (such as writing this book), we have the most vibrations running through our brain, and this frequency is called gamma. Perhaps this is an indication that the largest part of our neural network is active and supporting our mental processes, although the research into this is still ongoing.

When we are awake and going about our daily business of living, such as driving to work, packing lunch for the kids, and making supper, we are in the next level of vibration called beta. This is characterized by mental activity that is alert, though it lacks the intense focus of gamma. And at the end of the long workday, as we lie in bed, just before we are actually asleep, we find the magic minutes called theta.

Theta is really important to our subconscious mind because scientists have discovered that it is the "music" that the subconscious mind moves to. When we begin to reprogram our minds, this is the soundtrack to the new movie that we want to make. Theta brainwaves bypass the encoding process and force new knowledge into the subconscious mind. Combining this with repetitive concepts such as words, images, sounds, and phrases like affirmations have the potential to create new information highways through our subconscious mind, thereby changing how we react to situations when we are awake. Sounds like brainwashing?

In a way, it is. Literally! It allows us to "wash" the brain, to repack that laundry basket of our mind, and stack the new, "cleaner" items on top, where we can get hold of it immediately before we rush out of the house. Though we can't erase the knowledge already in our subconscious mind, we can rewrite the Search Engine Optimization (SEO) of our mind's Internet. We can force our subconscious mind to choose that which we have added during theta brain waves when it does the next mind search in response to outside stimuli from our senses.

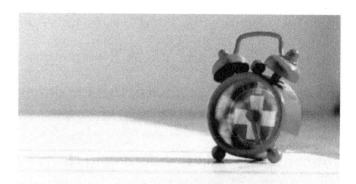

Gamma: 32-100 Hz

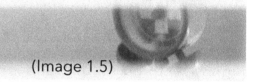

(Image 1.5)

This state of mind is the most alert, and we use it when we are engaged in mentally taxing activities such as studying or learning new knowledge (Image 1.5)

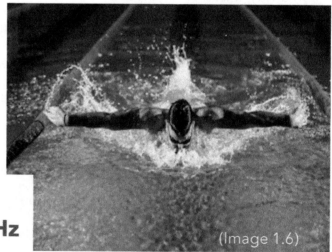

(Image 1.6)

Beta: 13-32 Hz

This is when we are alert, but relaxed. We can do routine activities such as playing sports, reading books, and tying our shoes during this state. (Image 1.6)

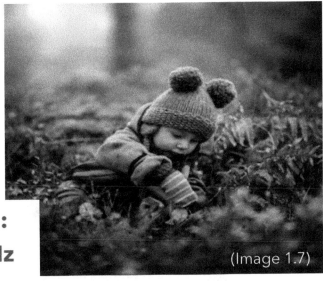

Alpha:
8-13 Hz

(Image 1.7)

Here we are relaxed, though not sleepy. This is when there are no demands being made of the brain, such as when we are busy showering, enjoying a quiet day outside, and engaging in soothing routines such as brushing our hair. (Image 1.7)

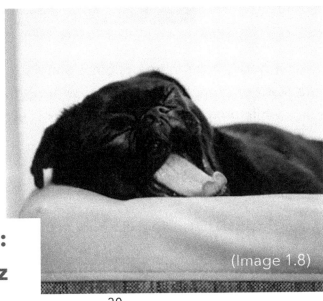

Theta:
4-8 Hz

(Image 1.8)

The magic minutes before we fall asleep. Our consciousness (which takes in outside stimuli) is reduced and we are in a state of suggestibility, almost like hypnosis. You slip into a state of easy dreaming, but not full sleep as yet. You will notice the yawn reaction happening spontaneously as your mind begins to "disconnect" and the subconscious opens to direct input. (Image 1.8)

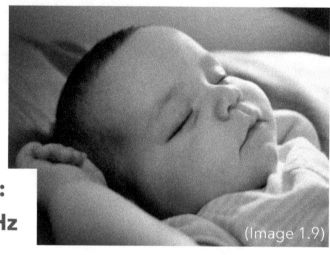

Delta: 0,5-4 Hz

(Image 1.9)

Our bodily awareness becomes almost zero, and we are in a state of complete relaxation, with no thoughts taking place while the body repairs itself. This is usually when cell production also increases. (Image 1.9)

Following this, it has been reasoned that by listening to music that plays at a specific frequency, we can stimulate our brains to enter the required state to be programmed.

Hence, music playing at 32-100 Hz is greatly beneficial when we are busy studying for exams. This theory has been proven with experiments using people who have epilepsy. If strobe lights or sound pulses are used to trigger the frequency that causes an epileptic fit, the test subjects all responded by having an epileptic reaction to those frequencies (Brainworks.com, n.d.). Brainwave entrainment has also become a booming industry, with sounds, music, and meditations being sold to improve memory, sleep, and relaxation.

The levels of consciousness and subconsciousness can certainly offer us a way to interact with and manipulate our minds. Many influential public figures such as actors, politicians, and business leaders have confessed to subscribing to the practice of managing their subconscious minds to program their minds and achieve their goals more effectively.

How Does the Subconscious Mind Work?

As previously stated, the subconscious mind becomes active at birth. When we are born, our mind is a blank slate that has nothing stored, except for a few inherited or inborn instincts (Stoycheva, 2019)[5]. We are instinctively afraid of the dark, animals, and heights. Just think of babies who cry when they are scared (which is often). This crying instinct is aimed at calling the protector (its mother or father) to come and defend the infant against damage or harm. As the child's mind develops, the subconscious mind also develops. It is a recording device that records EVERYTHING. There really seems to be no filter to stop it from recording the world around it. The subconscious mind is hardwired into our senses, so it records everything we see, hear, smell, touch, and taste. It also records events, results, and feelings. Basically, it is a giant sponge for our lives.

---

[5]Stoycheva, V. (2019). Hack Your Unconscious: Why Negative Feelings Linger Part I: Three reasons why negative emotions get you so worked up.

Over time, we are exposed to certain information bits that are repetitive in nature. We might hear our dad say that we are lazy, we don't make him proud, and we will be failures. We might also hear our mother cheering us on at the football match, screaming when we are playing well, but become quiet or even rebuking us when we don't play well. In either case, these all go into the subconscious mind, where it becomes recorded as a pattern of thought. Our recorded words, images, sounds, values, and even traumatic memories all together form our habitual guides to behavior. This is not an actual user-manual like you get with your TV (which you anyways don't look at). It is like being directed by something you can't see, hear, or even speak of.

We are unconscious of the subconscious' directives. But, instinctively, and without even knowing we do so, we respond to the subconscious directives we are given. If you were the child in the above scenario, you would immediately react with negativity to failure since it was frowned upon during your formative years. Within your mind, sucked up within the vast expanses of our subconscious mind, there is a program that has been created using this information. According to Lipton (2019) it plays non-stop and tells your mind (all without you knowing) that you are not worthy. That only in winning, getting a promotion at work, or succeeding in everything and being the best you can you be, will you show your worth. It is what your years of programming since childhood have been recording, and your subconscious mind believes it.

Sadly, we are much better at recording events and information that has a negative undertone since our instinctual brain believes it relates to self-preservation (Stoycheva, 2019). When something that is loaded with our stronger and more primitive emotions such as fear, anger, and lust occurs, we tend to place those at the top of the list in our subconscious mind. These will then be the first to be retrieved as memories or be most likely to be turned into habituated patterns of behavior. Incidentally, this is probably why we tend to be aggressive drivers. We may not have started out that way, but driving can be a high-stress task, which often involves negative emotions such as fear ("Oh, God, that car's going to hit me!") and anger ("You idiot! You can't just park there!"). With enough stressful events programmed into our memories, our subconscious mind will quickly kick into fight or flight mode, select an aggressive behavior program, and act accordingly. While you are driving, your subconscious mind is sending you a "download" that runs in the background (remember, you are not consciously aware of it) and this message is: "Be careful, be alert, be prepared, defend your lane, the other drivers are idiots and the enemy." Small wonder that road rage is becoming an epidemic, and almost half of all drivers have experienced it themselves as either the aggressor or victim, according to Jean Lawrence (WebMD.com, n.d.).

When trying to place a memory or thought higher up in the subconscious mind's search program, it is unfortunate that the subconscious mind pays much more attention to emotionally laden information and extremely negative feedback. Stoycheva (2019) continues this reasoning by stating that this is why sex and violence sell and is also why we see so much of it in the media and the entertainment industry. Since these are the things that drove primitive humans, it makes perfect sense. It seems then that the subconscious mind is drawn to information that promotes survival. As mentioned previously, the subconscious mind also controls the automated processes in the body, such as respiration and digestion, and it is always trying to maintain the balance or congruence between the internal world (of the mind) and the external world (of the body) (Lipton, 2019). Therefore, it can be said that the subconscious mind works to maintain our survival (through our baser instincts) while also maintaining a homeostatic balance within our bodies to the outside world.

So, if you are feeling aggressive because you are driving (and your subconscious mind is playing track 101 road aggression on its playlist), your subconscious mind will also trigger your mind into releasing more adrenaline (just in case you have to actually fight the other drivers for survival). Your feelings or emotional state is, therefore, matched to the physical level of alertness by your subconscious mind. Soon, your feelings (or more accurately, the subconscious mind's feelings) become habits that you don't even think about or question. The subconscious mind then works to control our responses to the world around us in a preprogrammed way that many of us are "blissfully" unaware of. By not questioning this system of operation, we are held back from achieving peace and inner happiness.

Boundaries of Consciousness

Here's a scary thought. (Now your subconscious mind will immediately direct your behavior to do this – you'll become afraid, cynical, or even deny it entirely.) Scientists don't actually know what anesthesia does! Yip. Most of us have had at least minor surgery in our lives, yet the doctors (whom we trust) aren't even sure what the drugs they administer do or how it "knocks us out" (Farrell, 2011)[6]. Of course, research into the boundaries of consciousness is still ongoing, and we will (hopefully) learn exactly what those drugs do and why some people struggle to regain their consciousness afterward. George Mashour, an anesthetist at the University of Michigan, is referenced (Farrell, 2011) as saying that scientists have discovered that anesthesia temporarily blocks the feedback of stimulus into the conscious mind, and thereby it prevents us from feeling

[6]Farrel, J. (2011). Neuroscientists Close in on the Boundaries of Consciousness.

38

anything during the surgery. However, it is still not clear what effect this has on the subconscious mind, which draws its information from more than just our pain receptors. Thus, the debate rages on about where the boundaries of consciousness can be drawn. Where is the point that humans "switch off," and what happens to the subconscious mind that doesn't switch off, ever?

"The boundary of the conscious mind is not fixed around the skin of the biological individual but is fragile and hard-won, and always open to negotiation," (Kiverstein & Kirchhoff, 2019)[7]. This means that our consciousness is more than the sum of our physical components. It is more than just our cells, the bundles of neurons, and the electrical impulses that carry thought. We are surrounded every day by people, things, situations, and emotional stimuli and these have an impact on our life experience or what gets coded into our subconscious mind, and these should be counted as part of that mind or consciousness. Hence, the people around us, where we live, our proximal environment, and daily stimuli also form part of our consciousness (and unconsciousness). Perhaps this is why motivational speakers often advise that people surround

---

[7]Kiverstein, J & Kirchoff, M. (2019). The Boundaries of the Conscious Mind.

themselves with positive people? The habits and attitudes of those we frequently interact with become stimuli that enter our subconscious mind, and these direct our conscious behavior. Our consciousness is, therefore, not limited by our brains but are rather defined by what and who we choose to associate with.

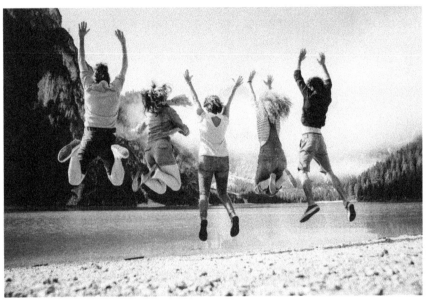

(Image 1.10)

By frequently associating with positive people, we internalize their positive stimulus into our subconscious minds. They become a part of our consciousness as we adopt a kind of group-think. (Image 1.10

So, "by your friends will you be judged" – as the saying goes. Naturalists have for hundreds of years studied the so-called "primitive" cultures of the world where group identity is not simply a cultural norm, but an actual part of the individual's consciousness. In parts of Africa where ancestor worship continues, the ancestors form a part of the consciousness, which is quite difficult to explain to the western world where the mainstream philosophy seems to be "me, myself, and I." As we learn about human consciousness, we will, in all likelihood, continue to expand the definitions regarding the boundaries of consciousness for it has certainly been a debate in religious circles for years.

Subconscious Patterns

We've all fallen into the habit of habit. That moment when we do something, not because we chose to, but because we are programmed to. One example that always has embarrassing results is the "hi" test. When you are at a social gathering, without being obvious, greet someone with only one word - "hi." When the other person returns the greeting, they will, in all likelihood, respond with "Hi, I'm fine, and you?" The subconscious mind has preprogrammed a greeting ritual that follows a certain

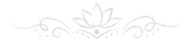

pattern. We don't always even listen to whether the other person had inquired about our health, yet we are preprogrammed with the response, "I'm fine, and you."

Our subconscious mind selects appropriate responses to outside stimuli. With repetitive responses, the mind programs these actions into the complex cognitive system of the subconscious, and habits are born. When someone is used to something, it becomes their habit or pattern according to which they operate. If someone is a habit-driven shopper, they will always buy the same products without even considering a new product or seeing a special on a different product. The same holds for the subconscious mind. If it chooses a habit to follow for a certain event (like taking the same route to work every day), it will not encourage deviation from this habit since deviation introduces new information that the subconscious is not familiar with. The subconscious mind will fight this disruption (which it sees as threatening) by throwing a temper tantrum in our mind. You may feel the effects of this in the form of emotions like rage or fear ("Road works? Why can't I drive there; I always drive there!") suddenly surging in your mind. Your subconscious

mind is so pattern-driven that it will block or override new stimuli that intrude upon its process. (You might not see or consider that there is a shortcut to work, and instead, you'll end up driving the same route every day.) If you are really honest, we've all had temper tantrums for no "apparent reason." You feel grumpy because...No, wait, you don't know why. However, your subconscious mind knows why. It's the one that gave you those emotions. These emotions are likely a response to stimuli that your mind is not happy to encode or new information that challenges its habits.

An example of a habit that we can all do without, but most of us have in common, is toxic thinking. This is when we have the habit of viewing a situation through a negative lens. Whatever happens, we believe that we will not be able to deal with it, and when someone else can deal with the challenge, we give in to jealousy, and as a result, we engage in negative self-talk. "Toxic thinking is self-perpetuating" (Staik, 2016). It cheats our brains into thinking that it has responded correctly with fear-driven behavior by creating a reward or validation for that behavior, and, therefore, we do more of the same harmful behavior. Hence, if you are faced with a challenging

43

situation such as competing for a promotion at work, you might habitually think that you don't stand a chance since you are not educated enough. (After all, you didn't get the previous promotion because of your inferior qualifications - which is the validation of the erroneous thinking.) If you don't get the job (again), your self-evaluation will reinforce this perception by motivating that the successful candidate had a degree, and you don't. (Can you hear your subconscious mind fueling negative self-talk like: "See, I just knew it. I'll never get anywhere since I'm not qualified or smart enough.") Your subconscious mind is already in the pattern of negativity, and it will not even allow you to take in alternative suggestions. (Maybe the other candidate got the promotion because they are friendlier or better spoken than you?)

Our subconscious mind is the real driver in our lives, and the reality is that we are really the co-pilot, not the other way around. But this need not be an adversarial relationship, and, in fact, the subconscious mind can be our best friend, staunchest supporter, and ever-present ally - it all depends on creating a useful perspective on life's events and our reactions to those events. Our mental states change as we encode more information, and our subconscious mind changes its perspective and storage system. In learning how to work with the subconscious mind, we can develop our assets and skills to reach our full potential and lead satisfying lives.

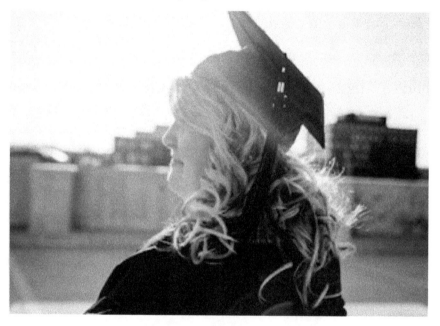

(Image 1.11)

Your subconscious mind will perpetuate emotionally laden views such as not being educated enough to further entrench behavioral thinking.

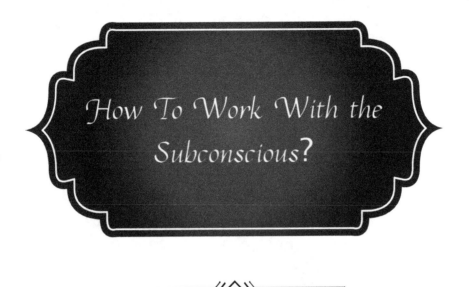

How To Work With the Subconscious?

Why would you want to work with the subconscious mind? It certainly seems like a scary and intimidating part of your brain, and one that you are possibly not prepared to work with. In a way, your brain is a little like Dr. Jekyll and Mr. Hyde. It has the conscious part that is logical and clear thinking like Dr. Hyde, while the subconscious mind is an emotional beast like Mr. Hyde. If we wish to reach our full potential in life and lead a peaceful and fulfilling existence, then we need to find a way to communicate with Mr. Hyde and bring him under control.

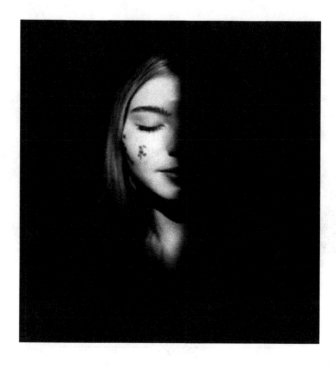

(Image 2.1)

We need to work with our subconscious mind to unify the dualities of our mind if we are to become successful and effective, fully functioning human beings. (Image 2.1)

Communication With the Subconscious

According to Lipton's blog (2017)[8], our subconscious minds are like computers that record and store our perceptions of the world around us. This information is

---

[8]Lipton, B. (2017). How to Heal Your Body With Your Mind.

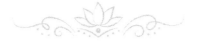

always available, even when this has been removed from context and should no longer be valid. It is always, therefore, playing our experiences back at us. So, if you want to tell your subconscious mind to stop smoking, for instance, it's the equivalent to scolding your screaming child, who shuts his ears and screams, "Lalalala!" If you want to communicate effectively with your subconscious mind, you need to find a way to get that "child" interested and speak at a level that they will understand. Any parent will know that we communicate with age appropriate language when we talk to young children. Likewise, we need to find the correct words and input mechanism to reach our little Mr. Hyde and bring him to the table for negotiations.

We have established in Part One that the brain and its state of wakefulness operate at specific frequencies that can trigger or reinforce that particular state of mind. Students who wish to study better would benefit from music ranging from 40 Hz to 100 Hz; however, the human ear is not capable of hearing effectively at this range. Mostly, it would sound like a deep bass noise, which is something that is felt more than heard – if you have good enough speakers, that is.

When you want to communicate with the subconscious mind, you need to dance to its beat, which happens to be at 3-8 Hz (Brainworks, n.d.). This is the natural state or brain frequency that occurs just before we fall asleep, and it is that magic step where the conscious mind pauses and the subconscious mind stops being "chatty" and starts to listen. This is the intersection in our minds where we can intentionally pre-plan to introduce information into our subconscious mind and know that the "child" will not be ignoring us. Since our conscious mind is then on the "snooze" function, we can't enter into a debate with our subconscious mind; however, we can prepare ahead of time with audio recordings, visualization, and meditations to get our message across.

Richards (2016)[9] also supports this science when he states that we are in a deep hypnotic state associated with theta brain waves from the last trimester of pregnancy to age seven. This is why children can combine reality with fantasy so easily (Lipton, 2019). Imagination becomes a

---

[9]Richards, C. (2016). Reprogramming Your Subconscious Mind. Retrieved

factor that we can then also use as a method of communication between our intentions (consciousness) and our habits (subconsciousness). Forming an effective communication strategy is vital to reprogramming our subconscious and rewriting its behavior programs that may no longer be in our best interests.

If you are wondering what would be the point of all this and it sounds way too much like geek-speak, then consider the following scenario:

Lisa comes from an abusive family, where, from an early age, her father used to tell her that she should be seen and not heard. (Sound familiar?) When Lisa did speak up about things she cared about, she was shut down by her distant parents, and she soon learned to keep her thoughts to herself and be pleasing to her "betters." Fast forward 20 odd years; Lisa is now an adult and she is desperately but secretly unhappy. She doesn't know why she just can't get promoted at work, and she feels that she is not valued. She has also entered yet another abusive relationship. Her boyfriend has now begun to beat her, and she doesn't know what to do about it. Even calling the police fills her with fear - What if they don't believe her? Lisa is a typical example of a person who is suffering from the programs playing in her subconscious mind.

Lisa's subconscious mind was programmed as a young child to replay a soundtrack that features the tracks, "I should be seen and not heard," "People are better than me, and I should do what makes them happy," and "No one will believe me, since I am not valued." If Lisa doesn't begin to connect her subconscious and her conscious minds, she will never realize that her subconscious mind has been leading her down a path she really doesn't want to be on. She doesn't get promoted at work, because her subconscious mind says, "Be seen, not heard," and she is in abusive relationships because her subconscious mind sees these abusive people (like her parents) as being part of a habit (known pattern of behavior) and, therefore, OK.

Once Lisa connects her conscious (reasoning mind) and subconscious (habit forming) minds, she will be able to embark on the road to healing. "As your perception changes, you change the message that your nervous system communicates to the cells of your body" (Lipton, 2017). This is vitally important for change to happen, as the programs of your subconscious mind runs 95% of the time. When Lisa sees her tape-recording-stuck-in-the-rut-of-the-past subconscious mind for what it is doing to her, she will be able to initiate change. Using the channel of communication that theta waves offer, combined with meditation (mindfulness), and visualizations, Lisa can begin to imagine new habits that will change her life for the better.

This is how she can create change through communication:

Current Program:	*"Other people are better than me, and I should make them happy."*
Results:	*Lisa accepts being passed over for promotion and believes she's to blame when her boyfriend is unhappy.*
New Program:	*"My joy is important, and I make others happy when I am happy."*
New Results:	*Lisa speaks up when she sees a promotion at work opening, and she is invited to apply, as the company values her. She begins asserting herself in her relationship, and believes that her happiness is also important*

Current Program:	*"I should be seen and not heard."*
Results:	*Lisa keeps quiet; she doesn't speak up for herself.*
New Program:	*"My opinion is valuable; people want to hear what I have to say."*
New Results:	*Lisa speaks up at work, participates in group discussions, and she is noticed by her bosses who start giving her more responsibilities and opportunities*

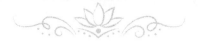

Current Program:	"No one believes me."
Results:	Lisa never speaks up when she feels upset; she believes that people will just make fun of her or think she's overreacting and seeking attention.
New Program:	"I believe in myself, and people who love me care about me."
New Results:	Lisa speaks out when she is unhappy. She speaks with authority and identifies when people value her, and she values herself.

Lisa would be able to communicate with her subconscious mind by using theta brain waves, meditation, visualization, and affirmations to create a much more pleasing set of habits in her mind. It is not possible to force the subconscious mind. Despite this, scientists have tried to use more unethical methods such as electroconvulsive therapy (ECT) to trick the subconscious mind into believing that the mind is healed. Barbaric treatments like this would be unnecessary if we would begin to communicate with the subconscious mind and make it our friend and ally, not our enemy and source of fear.

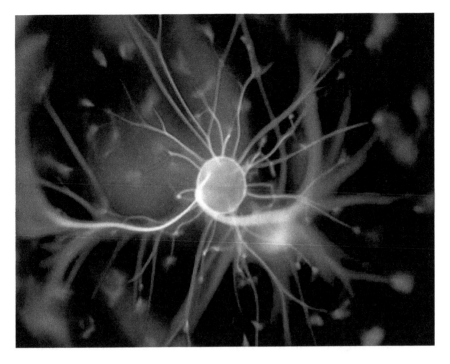

(Image 2.2)

Communicating with our subconscious mind and achieving lasting change to damaging routines or patterns of behavior is a far better strategy than more invasive methods like ECT and chemically numbing our subconscious mind with antidepressants. (Image 2.2)

Subconscious Answers

Up until now, we have said that the conscious mind is the logical center and that we use it to solve problems since we are also imaginative beings, and problem-solving is part of daily life. At some point in life, you will be trying to solve a vexing problem and hitting a blank, when suddenly a solution seems to appear as if magically in your mind. If you take a moment to consider where that solution came from, you can thank your subconscious mind. The subconscious mind is the big gun that we take out when we need to use maximum power to solve a problem or fight a challenge. In computer terms, the subconscious mind is like a huge several terabyte hard drive versus a much smaller USB drive. It has an immeasurable capacity, and it can multitask like a boss!

According to Birch (2018), our subconscious mind is much more powerful than our conscious mind, and it can deal with a great deal more data in the form of our thoughts, events we experience, and our emotions, as well as dealing with the myriad of processes involved in our thinking and keeping our body running. This means that your subconscious mind can reach conclusions based upon infinitesimal possibilities that your conscious mind could never have processed or even considered. Plainly put, your subconscious has abilities that verge on being superpowers! It can identify connections, make deductions, and create new rhythms of thought that we could never accomplish without this incredible part of our mind.

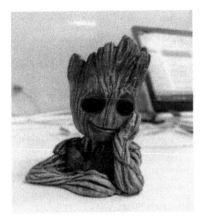

Like Baby Groot, we are all busy learning about our incredible and unexplored abilities as we develop them. We learn to make full use of the subconscious mind through solving problems, and through it, helping us reach our goals. (Image 2.3)

On a daily basis, we are faced with challenges and problems that need solving and intervention. The subconscious mind is really great at both these things, but, at times, it doesn't seem to be a cooperative partner. In fact, it's absent most of the time when we think we need it. (The minute that we think we need it, we are using our conscious mind, and this blocks out the subconscious mind since their brain waves don't match.) We have already hinted at the fact that communicating with the subconscious mind is not as simple as sending it an email. However, apart from enlisting its help through the lengthy processes of theta meditations and visualizations (which we'll discuss in more detail later), we can also post a notice on the mind's community board, so to speak. We can do this by accumulating as much information as possible about our problem.

"The more conscious information you stuff into the back-office of your subconscious [the more it] forces your brain [to] acknowledge the problem as a priority, and [the encoding process] adds that issue to your subconscious queue" (Birch 2018)[10]. Hence, reading about your problem, talking about it, discussing it with others, and consciously pursuing solutions relating to the main problem is like pelting your subconscious mind with rocks to get its attention. The trick is that when the subconscious mind has taken note and found a solution, we are often not listening to hear the answer.

Previously, we created the analogy of the subconscious mind being like the child who screams "Lalala!" when the parent wants to talk to it. And just like that neglected and poorly socialized child, the subconscious mind also throws

---

[10]Birch, A. (2018). How to Engage Your Subconscious Mind to Solve Your Toughest Problems.

a little hissy fit when it is trying to talk to its parent, but the parent is too busy to listen. It stamps its foot and hides in a corner. For us to be able to hear the answers that the subconscious mind has created, we need to listen. Not with our ears, not with our thoughts, but by quieting our minds. We need to stop worrying about the problem and wait. Yes, just wait. And it doesn't take as long as you fear it will for you to receive an answer from your subconscious mind. Truly, it's quite eager to share its brilliance with us, but it doesn't like the competition that the conscious mind offers (like a kind of sibling rivalry) and, therefore, if we can quiet down the conscious mind, we encourage our brain to turn to the lower frequencies like theta and delta where we can hear the subconscious better. Birch (2018) recommends that we find time to sit without thinking, while Julia Cameron (renowned author and self-help mentor) recommends that we take 20-minute walks to disconnect our conscious mind by doing a routine activity that falls into the subconscious domain and activates the appropriate brain waves.

Rock (2012)[11] discusses the research of neuroscientist professor David Cresswell where it was found among test subjects who all faced problems that those who thought about the problem non-stop for a while often reached an incorrect solution, while the others who had to answer immediately did not do well either. The last group was given a distractor task, such as coloring in a picture that doesn't require active thought, after they were presented with the problem. This last group reached the most correct and complete solutions to the problem, despite having seemingly not spent much time on the problem at all. Rock also points out that the distractor task does not have to be of any significant length, so it will not require an intense meditation or a night of sleep to reach a solution. Perhaps this is why adult coloring books have become quite popular today? Small-scale activities that temporarily quiet the conscious mind, such as coloring, knitting, and showering, all allow the subconscious the opportunity to pass its solutions on to us, like magic! Remember, the

---

[11]Rock, D. (2012). Stop Trying To Solve Problems: Hack the brain to increase complex problem solving.

subconscious mind is the director of routing activities, and we can use these to draw it out.

Finally, there is a technique, kind of like a human Ouija board, that is believed to be a way to directly communicate with the subconscious mind with simple "yes" and "no" responses. This is still quite theoretical, though the science behind it is based on fact. It's called Muscle Testing or Applied Kinesiology. It is based on the science of electrical impulses or energy that we have in our bodies (because, like in *The Matrix*, human bodies are basically large-scale batteries with an energy charge). Theoretically, that energy can respond according to the wishes of the subconscious mind since it controls all bodily processes. The senses are also hard-wired into the subconscious mind, endlessly feeding it information to be recorded. Scher (2019)[12] writes that events and emotions can overload the electrical system of our bodies temporarily, causing a momentary weakness that can cause our muscles to move involuntarily (in other words, our muscles move on the instruction of the subconscious mind, not our conscious desire). Getting the

[12]Scher, A. (n.d.). Muscle Testing: Getting Answers From the Subconscious Mind.

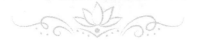

answers involves what is called a "sway test." The test subject taps their thymus gland (just below where your chin would reach if you tucked it onto your chest) for 30 seconds. Questions are then asked (these questions must have a "yes" or "no" answer), and the body will "sway" forward for positive answers and backward for negative answers. So, if your problem is something like, "Is my approach to winning new contracts working?" your body would sway backward if your subconscious mind believes that your current strategy is not working. Muscle Testing may be a bit far off the beaten path and possibly fall more in the category of pseudo-science, but it is still interesting in its approach of letting our subconscious mind help in solving our problems.

The subconscious mind wants to share its incredible insights with us, and it wants to impress us and make our lives better. Despite it having the tendency to generate negative habits and routines, it is capable of being a force for good. It simply requires that there are open channels of communication, both to "ask" questions and "receive" answers.

How to Teach the Brain to Filter Thoughts

"You suck!", "What's the point of that; I'm going to fail anyways?", "She's too pretty, and I'll never be noticed by that cute guy!", and "My boss doesn't like me" are all examples of negative self-talk. These depressing and often debilitating words are generated by our subconscious mind and they replay ad infinitum in our minds until we believe that we are not good enough and that we will never reach our goals. James (2016), contributing editor at Inc.com, writes that the subconscious mind has inherited survival instincts through our evolutionary development. It's a primitive defense mechanism that we are stuck with, despite us no longer needing to be on the fearful look out for predators. Today, these negative conversations that we have with ourselves bring us down and threaten our success in life.

Self-help author, Martha Beck (2008), refers to this as the fears of "lack and attack" where our primitive self will kick in and send us negative messages that derail our efforts. The negative self-talk above can each be drawn to a primitive fear that the subconscious mind is trying to keep you safe from.

Negative Self-Talk	Primitive Fear That Generates It
"You suck!"	*Popularity ensured that procreation could take place and that you would not be kicked out of the tribe. Being solitary meant death in the wild.*
"What's the point of that; I'm going to fail anyways?"	*Primitive man had a constant struggle for food and resources; wasting either threatened their future. They had to succeed without wasting energy or else they would starve.*
"She's too pretty, and I'll never be noticed by that cute guy!"	*Competition is as old as mankind. Jealousy is based on fearing that we would not be selected or taken care of, and we would not find a mate.*
"My boss doesn't like me."	*In primitive times, conflict was as commonplace as today. If the tribe leader didn't approve of you, chances were that you'd be eliminated soon. Fear itself can be equally threatening.*

However, today, many of these threats have been eliminated. You are not very likely to face a giant mammoth or saber-tooth cat in the city. Subconsciously, your mind is still alert and looking for these dangers. In combining information and assigning values based on the emotional reaction to that information, our subconscious mind is easily convinced that the boss, whom we may not like and also fear, is the new giant mammoth in your life. Consciously, we know that a boss is merely a stressed person, who is trying to increase productivity so that they don't have to fire staff. But subconsciously, our mind has decided that the boss is the mammoth, ready to bore you to death with their tusks. It is up to your conscious mind, and its logical faculties, to convince your subconscious mind that some information it receives is not threatening and does not need to be prioritized as being of life-saving importance. Only in filtering out the thoughts associated with negative information encoding can the patterns of behavior (like running from the mammoth-boss or fearing that colleague who gets all the promotions because he is a saber tooth tiger who will eat his competition) be changed. Sadly, since bad experiences or bad information activates our subconscious mind's survival instinct, these tend to stick quickly or enter the subconscious mind the easiest while positive experiences are not essential to keep us alive (according to the subconscious mind) and are, therefore, not prioritized.

There are a few techniques for snapping the subconscious mind back from running along the survival instinct ruts that it makes. These ruts tend to create negative thoughts, but with awareness and preparation, we can filter out negativity and increase our absorption of positive information, thereby creating new and constructive paths in the mind.

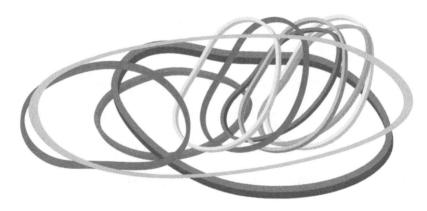

(Image 2.4)

Techniques such as using an elastic band on your wrist, which you flick every time you think a negative thought, reverses the subconscious mind's survival instincts - it will change behavior that results in physical pain. (Image 2.4)

Filtering out negative thoughts may not be easy for everyone, especially when you are already lacking a high self-esteem. You may be too intimidated to question others when they "talk down" at you and much more so when you have to face your own negativity. Wilding (2016)[13] writes in *Forbes Magazine* that you may feel like you do not deserve success and, as a result, start with negative self-talk or self-sabotaging thoughts that will run you down to a level your own, poorly developed self-esteem might find acceptable. She suggests that it may be a better approach to acknowledge thoughts that limit us rather than trying to replace them or deny them. If a certain thought is self-challenging such as "I am a failure," it is better to "air" that thought out and evaluate it with your critical reasoning faculties. Once a negative thought has been evaluated and its validity debunked through careful reasoning, such as contradicting it with evidence in line of "I have completed a degree. I am successful at work. I have a loving family," that negative thought loses its power, and it is less likely to crop up again.

It all boils down to who is in control of our thoughts. Initially, our subconscious minds are the autopilots to our

---

[13]Wilding, M. (2016). Forget Positive Thinking: This Is How To Actually Change Negative Thoughts For Success.

lives, but the more we flick that switch to become self-responsible and self-aware, the more we will be able to if not control our thoughts, then at least monitor and participate in them.

Meditation

Our lives are stressful existences, often driven by unrealistic fears that cascade from our subconscious mind, which evaluates everything around us in terms of "fight or flight." Sadly, the more stressed we are, the more our subconscious mind believes that it is correct in reacting negatively so that it can keep us alive (by running from the metaphorical tigers). Greenberg (2011) writes that meditative practices, as well as other non-invasive techniques like herbs and movement therapies (like tai chi), can be useful to bring the "mind back into balance"; while Mayer (2018) believes that meditation can bring a specific mental balance. Mayer also explains that during meditation (or mindfulness), the brain waves are lowered to within the bandwidth of theta, which is, of course, where we can begin making suggestions to our subconscious mind. This is where saying things like, "be more positive" or "please, look at this possibility" find their way into the wonderful factory of our mind where we encode our habits.

So, how does meditation work? Mayer suggests five steps for introducing beginners to meditation. These steps are really easy, and most of us will achieve a moderately successful meditation on the first attempt. Here are a few basic steps:

•*First step of meditation: Focus*

The first step is about focusing your mind onto something that is, in a word, boring. It needs to be an object that is unchanging and easily seen. This is perhaps why the Buddhists have traditionally focused their minds using beads due to their round and unchanging shapes. Using your mind, observe the shape of the object you have chosen. If your attention wanders, just gently bring it back to the shape, focusing on the roundness of the bead (for instance). This is how, without intending to, you create a kind of stillness in your mind, because the simplistic object you have chosen does not require analysis or reaction. It simply is.

Some other induction techniques might focus on your body parts, slowly focusing on one particular part and then moving on to the next when the part has begun to feel relaxed. Shakti Gawaine[14], one of the best-renowned visualization practitioners, refers to focusing on the light between your eyes and letting that light expand outwards to encompass the whole of your mind, bringing calm emptiness with it. These techniques might sound a bit too new-age to some, and they can certainly be more difficult at the beginning (when I try to focus on my body parts, I tend to fixate on how less than perfect they are!). But they are certainly worth exploring while you look for the method that works best for you. I have even heard of people who draw repetitive shapes and focus on the area where the pen meets the page, like a form

---

[14]Staik, A. (2016). The Neuroscience of Changing Toxic Thinking Patterns (1 of 2). Retrieved on: 11.15.2019 from

of mandala creation. Whatever works will be up to each individual's preference.

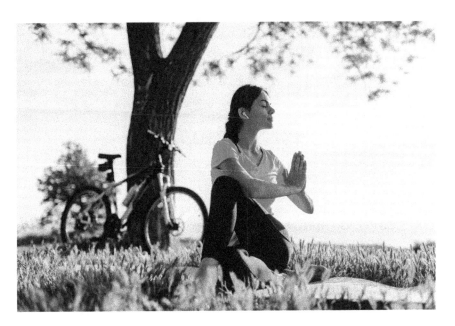

(Image 2.5)

As with all things in life, the more we practice it, the better we will get at it. Even if you don't reach theta brain waves in your first try at meditation, it will still lower your brain waves (perhaps down to delta or alpha), where we are in a more relaxed mental state, which is also beneficial to our health. (Image 2.5)

•Second step of meditation: Access an idea or belief that you want to change

Instead of fighting with that idea, believe that this applied to you before, but it no longer does, and begin to visualize how you see this belief changing going forward in life. So, if you have a belief of "I am not the brightest penny," then you can accept that maybe you were not first in line when IQ was handed out; however, you were right at the front when they handed out aptitude and you are hardworking and talented. Your belief might be visualized as changing to "I am a hard worker, and I never give up."

•Step three of meditation: Observe the change you want to be

While you are in this suggestive state, where the conscious mind is barely present and the subconscious mind is also at the table for negotiations, you can begin to visualize yourself entering a dialogue with yourself. In psychological terms, human beings always move from the known to the unknown. Therefore, it is a good idea to begin by visualizing yourself according to the limiting belief at first (painful as that may be) and then move to the new way you want to be. So, you might start by seeing how you failed tests in the *past due to not being smart enough. From this point on, you shift your perspective. You see yourself putting in the hard work, not giving up, and eventually passing that exam that you need to pass; in other words, you move to the unknown – the new you.*

•Step four of meditation: Voice the change

We often hear that people struggle to find their inner voice. It's probably because of all the negative self-talk that drowns out your voice. With mindfulness and meditation, you can begin to find that inner voice again. Find a way to express the change you want by phrasing it into a short but powerful sentence or mantra. In your visualization, you see yourself as being the hardworking academic underachiever, but you can give yourself a motto to live by, such as "I am an inspiration to other students, because I never give up." Your visualization then changes, and you see yourself as being an inspiration to other students and getting together to form study groups. In the end, this will result in your academics also improving due to your hard work and the involvement of your peers.

•*Step five of meditation: Balance want and desire*

Your two minds must be in agreement with each other's wishes. The subconscious mind wants to keep you safe; that's why it creates routines that it sees as being protective of your survival. So, you feel road rage because your subconscious mind sees driving as a dangerous task where the introduction of extra brain chemistry to raise your level of alertness is beneficial. The extra adrenaline and testosterone stimulate your attention and physical readiness (to run from that tiger or fight off that rival from the other tribe) while also making you more aggressive as a side-effect. Your conscious mind wants to be at peace with your fellow humans while driving safely, and with as little stress as possible, to work in the morning. When planning your meditative visualization or affirmations in this case, it is a good idea to keep both your minds happy. You might start by creating thoughts or behavior patterns like *"I am a good driver, and I arrive safely and happily at my destination."*

If you are still not sure about this notion of creating the thoughts you desire with meditation, then perhaps you should consider the research done on the topic. A research study in 2003 by scientist Richard Davidson (Greenberg, 2011) indicated that the participants showed significant changes in the electrical activity of their brains over eight weeks. The participants also had a better immune response to the flu after they had received the meditation training, indicating that meditation even has benefits for our health. It really is a case of "think healthy, become healthy."

Rules of Conduct in Meditation

Meditation can be a really difficult habit to acquire. Yes, it should be a habit, not a once-off let's-try-it-and-see. If you were to go to the gym once in a while, you certainly wouldn't expect to build rock hard abs or lose 10 pounds. Likewise, it is illogical to expect lasting change to your mental habits if you only meditate or visualize once in a while. Remember, those negative thoughts and destructive patterns of behavior that are programmed to play in your subconscious mind are playing non-stop. You have to get ahead of that train if you hope to catch and stop it. For beginners, it's useful to consider the following rules to guide you on this new inclusion to your life. (And before you say, "I don't have time to start staring at a bead in the morning," you may be pleased to hear that the time is not wasted, but rather invested. If you invest that time, it will give you a lovely return - with compound interest and making you use time more efficiently.)

So, here are the basic rules of meditation (Eisler, 2015)[15]:

•Be comfortable

Sitting in clothes that are tight and uncomfortable will be painful and distracting. It's a good idea to be relaxed (and not have to worry about your pants riding down, exposing your plumber's crack) while you are trying to meditate in the cubicle at work during lunch. Try to find an environment where you will be comfortable. It doesn't have to be a local Hindi temple or Catholic church –this is not a religious experience (although, for some, it will soon begin

---

[15]Eisler, M. (2015). 10 Rules for New Meditators. s.

to feel like that due to the relief and sense of peace that it brings). You may feel comfortable sitting on the couch at home or in your car at work (in the parking lot and not driving!).

•Be alert

Strangely, it is important to be alert during meditation. This is possibly because the brain waves of deep sleep and our subconscious minds are very close to each other on the scale. The difference between delta and theta brain waves is not large at all. However, sleeping would negate much of the reconstructive work that you want to do on your belief systems.

•Time it

When you begin with any physically strenuous activity, you don't start out with unrealistic expectations. On your first day at the gym, you don't start with 50 push-ups (certainly, most of us would not survive that amount of exertion). The same holds true for meditation. When you start, it's best to start small (Cody, 2017)[16]. Instead of trying to be a meditative virtuoso, you can rather focus on five quality minutes a day for the first couple of days. When it

---

[16]Cody, S. (2017). 6 Ways to Get the Most From Meditation.

feels more comfortable, you can extend this to cover more aspects of meditation. It may seem like you are sitting there doing nothing, but in the beginning, it might be the hardest thing you've ever "done."

•Do it on the go

Life is busy! Many of us rush from one activity to the next, and we never seem to have even a minute to ourselves. The thought of finding five minutes or longer in the morning might be too overwhelming, creating a recipe for quitters. Rather, find the moments in between to start with. This might be the two minutes that you spend on the bathroom in the morning. You might multi-task and also meditate (instead of browsing Facebook on your mobile). Or you could meditate when you are waiting in the elevator for a stuffy five-minute trip up to the 40th floor. If you wait for opportunities to occur, you will never get started; however, if you go look for the time to be mindful, you will find it.

•Don't judge

This second last rule is the most important, according to Eisler (2015). We easily run ourselves down when we try something new. This is the doorway to doubt. DON'T do it!

It is not about judging or evaluating whether the meditation is working for you or not. When it starts working, you will know it. You will see the changes that you seek appearing in your life. If you feel that it is not working for you, the chances are that you have not managed to focus on that single image or object to the point of distraction. Remember, you need that sense of distraction to create an environment where your conscious mind is less loud and your subconscious stops babbling long enough to listen to you.

•Using technology

There is a wide variety of meditation facilitating devices and apps that are designed to help the new initiate explore meditation and in reaching their meditation goals. Though these might seem like wonderful tools to take the "hard work" out of "doing nothing," and they certainly serve a purpose, the importance of making that personal connection to your subconscious mind cannot be emphasized enough. Technology might get you the audience with your mind, but it's up to you to decide on what to say to it.

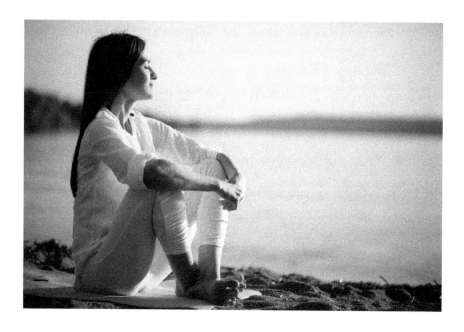

(Image 2.6)

Meditation can be as simple as sitting in a quiet place, closing your eyes, and listening to your breathing. One breath, two breaths, three breaths... (Image 2.6)

Lastly, it is interesting to point out that meditation, and the development of our minds, go hand-in-hand. Whether you want to use meditation, positive thinking, or hypnosis, we need a method to start talking to the best asset at our disposal - our subconscious mind. Hrala (2016) writes that meditation makes us more aware of our own subconscious actions or our "unawareness" and that this stimulates feelings of greater self-control. That "self" in self-control is greatly determined by our subconscious mind. If we want to change and improve ourselves, then we have to change our "self," we have to change our subconscious mind.

Our subconscious mind has tremendous power and processing capacity at its disposal, and if we can learn to work with it effectively, there is no telling how far in life we can go. The phrase "being a co-creator" of your life may seem a bit clichéd, but the reality is that no one should create our lives, except us (and God and the universe). If we allow the events and people in our lives to program our subconscious mind for us, we will be the ones to suffer. Your subconscious mind is a bit like an unruly teenager, but with effort, open channels of communication, and encouragement (as well as making sure that your teenager doesn't have druggie and alcoholic friends), we can help develop a top achiever that we can be proud of.

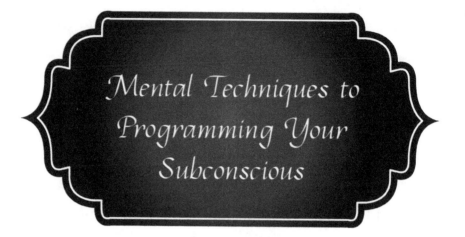

Mental Techniques to Programming Your Subconscious

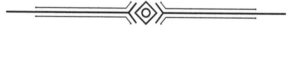

Many self-help gurus refer to us as having an inner child, which is supposed to be this pure and innocent side to ourselves. It is supposed to be creative, spiritual, and encouraging. Perhaps it is true. However, for most of us, the only child we have inside us is a screaming ADHD toddler who is hyperactive, never sleeps, feels that the world is against them, and that none of their friends want to play. That child is your subconscious mind. That child needs to be taught right from wrong, and they need to be raised to become well-functioning individuals within society (your mind). True, this child that we have inside us is creative, and they can come up with the most amazing solutions to problems if we let them. But every child needs a parent. You need to parent your subconscious mind (your inner child) and ensure that this child shares a belief system that you approve of. If this is not done, then your subconscious mind will begin to dictate what you do, how you do it, and how you feel about life. It decides these things based upon baser needs, such as your perceived safety, nutrition, and the reproduction of the species. Though this may have been fine and well during our early primitive times, it is no longer how we want to live our lives.

In the past, we used to silence the subconscious mind's patterns and behaviors to achieve a state of relative calm by using drugs and invasive "therapies." This theory of "shut it up" has in recent years become largely debunked. People no longer want their subconscious mind to be silenced; instead, they want to give it a voice and establish negotiations with it, making the subconscious mind your friend, not an enemy. The power of the subconscious mind is an amazing force that, if used correctly, can unleash our full potential and help us to achieve our goals through

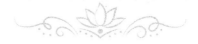

ingenuity and information processing at a level that our conscious minds can, as yet, not reach.

So, where does the concept of programming your subconscious mind fit in then? If we want to "negotiate" with our subconscious mind, how can we force it to do things a certain way? And that is where the confusion occurs. Words like "mind control," "programming techniques," and "methods" have been given a bad rep due to their abuse in the past. Modern-day approaches are much more moderate and inclusive than before. Your subconscious mind is included in the process, and it becomes your partner. In fact, the programming process is something that the subconscious mind already does every day by accepting and filing new information - you will now simply be selecting what you let your mind digest. It's sort of like a diabetic, who goes on a diet that supports their health (sugary sweets are not a good idea, but they can choose to eat healthily, although, they do sneak a treat now and again).

Now that you feel less guilty (or terrified) about reprogramming your subconscious mind, let's look at some techniques that are beneficial and fun, which will make a friend of your mind.

Imagination Is More Important Than Knowledge

This famous quote by Albert Einstein, a famous scientist, philosopher, and creator of the atomic theory, was recorded in 1929 when Einstein was talking about his life in an interview with *The Saturday Evening Post*. What is less well known is the second part of the quote - "For knowledge is limited, whereas imagination encircles the world," and this is where our subconscious mind comes into play. Our subconscious mind has a finite amount of knowledge (determined by our experiences and our sensory intake), yet it can solve any problem, no matter what. Through the infinite amount of associations that your subconscious mind can form from the information you have stored, it can tackle any issue and find a multitude of possible outcomes to that problem. This is one of the least understood aspects of the subconscious mind - it can be useful and positive when it is trained to work with the conscious mind.

Imagination is something that happens when your subconscious mind sends out a "random" series of memories or extrapolations to feed our conscious or logical mind; conclusions are reached, giving us imagination (or problem-solving). According to Earthsky.org (n.d.), imagination is where (when) the conscious mind "consciously manipulates images, symbols, ideas, and theories," and then creates the mental focus necessary to find solutions to issues and invent new thoughts about things. The brain (or mind) solves these problems by reorganizing the mind (our information). Andreasen (2011)[17] believes that the mind is a system that creates new file-codes on an ongoing basis, like the root system on a computer. It decides what information is important based on our values, emotions, experiences, and conscious decisions. In layman's terms, the subconscious mind looks for connections between different memories

---

[17] Andreasen, N.C. (2011). A Journey into Chaos: Creativity and the Unconscious.

and ideas. It then creates a range of possible answers or solutions to our problems.

An example of this would be if you need to decide what to wear for a Halloween party at work. Your subconscious mind would reference all the previous Halloween parties you have ever been to or seen. It would consider themes within the general idea of dress up parties, such as pirates, *Arabian Nights*, *Jungle Book*, and hospital themes. It would then use the information about what you have in your closet, consider how you could begin combining outfits (and even what it knows your friends have available for you to borrow). In the end, it will give your conscious mind some options, such as combining your black evening dress with biker boots and a leather jacket to create a gothic vampire look, or your white mini skirt with a sexy top and folding a white hat to play nurse. It would then be up to your conscious mind to decide on which imaginative option would be best received in your work environment. If your boss is very religious, they might not enjoy the vampire look (and you can put the ketchup back in the fridge). During these negotiations between your subconscious mind and the conscious mind, information is being exchanged both ways. You might end up adapting the nurse's look to rather become a nerdy scientist instead - since you know that your boss likes science, and you believe that impressing them will open future promotional opportunities for you.

Earlier, we indicated that the subconscious mind is in charge of maintaining balance. A challenge or problem creates tension in the body (and mind), which is not beneficial to the continued existence of the body. Hence, the subconscious mind sees problems (and their tensions) as a threat, and it will take the necessary steps to remedy the situation and protect the body (and mind). This is something that we can begin to consciously manipulate. If we continue with the Halloween scenario above, and one of your colleagues has been harassing you repeatedly at work or making you feel threatened, then your subconscious mind's creativity will be directed at protecting your survival. You might end up coming up with excuses not to attend that Halloween party, instead of thinking about costume possibilities. Your subconscious mind will be trying to remove you from the proximity of the fear-inducing person (your lecherous colleague), and this then takes precedence over the need to impress the bosses and win promotion.

Your subconscious mind is a "picture" brain. It sees solutions before your conscious mind can articulate them. If you were to be stranded on an island in the middle of the ocean, and you have only a pen, a box of dental floss, and a pair of ladies pantyhose... (did you start thinking of a solution?) Without even completing the scenario, your subconscious mind had already sent through a mass of associations to your conscious mind, which considered the practicalities and came up with a possible solution. It realized in mere milliseconds that you would be hungry on this island, and it also realized that it could use the pen's cap tied to the dental floss to make a hook and line, while the pantyhose could be used to make a fishing net, to catch the smaller fish. This scenario also indicates how your subconscious mind assigned priority to your survival. It didn't think that you could use the dental floss to bind the leaves of the palm trees into a book (or make paper pulp with the pantyhose) and then write your memoirs with the pen. That is not related to your survival, and, therefore, it is not ranked at the top of your subconscious mind's "Google

Search." In terms of the mind, it is not about what you would want, but rather about how you use what you know to sustain your continued existence.

This is not mere hearsay either, and scientists continue to investigate how our subconscious mind makes associations and uses those associations to reach conclusions. Neuroimaging studies have found evidence that people who are very creative experience increased brain activity in the areas connected with the making of associations when they are busy with tasks that involve finding solutions through associations (Andreasen, 2011). If those association cortices were blank, our subconscious mind would not be able to find a possible conclusion. It is the putting together of information (and forming neural pathways or thinking paradigms) that gives us creativity. We have to motivate our subconscious mind to search for alternative solutions and not simply jump to the first possible option (track 101 of the mind's playlist).

So, how did the first person to make a pair of scissors, for instance, decide that putting two pieces of metal that are only moderately sharpened would give us a tool that can cut fabric in a straight line? While creativity may not be the mother of invention, necessity certainly is. In our island scenario above, the urgency (of having to eat to survive) is instrumental in motivating the subconscious mind to find a solution.

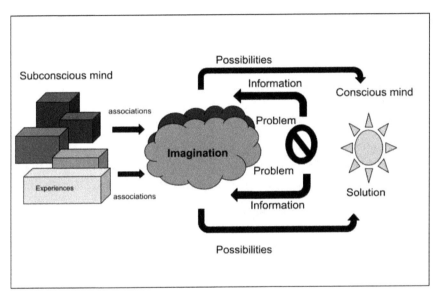

Flow of imagination. (Figure 3.1)

In Figure 3.1, we can clearly see the process of creativity or imagination explained. Your subconscious mind contains a wealth of stored up experiences, memories, and a gazillion other random facts and information bits. When a problem occurs, your conscious mind makes your subconscious mind aware of this (your senses also send information through and, at times, your subconscious mind knows there's a problem before your conscious mind even does). Your subconscious mind will begin the process of forming associations. Psychologists often use association tests to do evaluations of their patients, and it is one of the few ways in which we can directly "see" where the subconscious mind is "at." Imagination will send these associations through to the conscious mind, which will select the most appropriate action to take to solve the problem. This is, in theory, how it works, but once we add emotions to the mix, everything seems to get befuddled. Usually, we are not stuck in such obvious scenarios as the island scenario above. Due to our confusion, we end up feeling out of sorts and upset. We don't know why we feel upset, and we just tend to lash out. By using association tests, such as saying a word that pops into your mind with the stimulus of a flashcard or saying something in response to the famous Rorschach test, psychologists can get a clear indication of where your subconscious mind is heading.

Your subconscious mind is the originator of imagination, due to the stored information it has and the associations it can make.

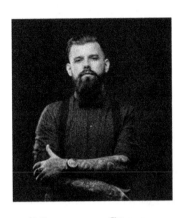

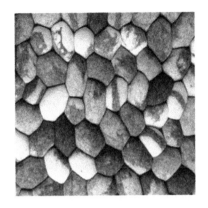

Man ➝ Strong   Rock ➝ Build

(Images 3.1)

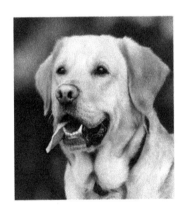

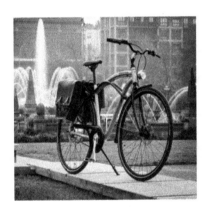

Dog ➝ Bark   Bicycle ➝ Travel

(Images 3.5)

Mind associations (Images 3.1 - 3.5)

Your subconscious mind does more than just suggest ideas to your conscious mind; it also takes action. Because your knowledge (which is kept in the subconscious mind) is based on past experiences, and the success or failure of our past actions, your subconscious mind is a bit of an expert at finding appropriate solutions, especially when it relates to your survival (just think of watching *MacGyver* on TV during the '80s or the new remake and all the incredible solutions that the character came up with -usually to save a life or to survive). A stimulated subconscious mind, which believes that it can find solutions, is an asset; however, a subconscious mind that has been subjected to mostly negative experiences (such as trauma) and has been conditioned to believe that it can't find solutions, will be in extreme survival mode. Cases where an abused woman stays with the abusive partner are prime examples of this. Their subconscious mind has been denied the positive past experiences to draw on to find a solution. Therefore, they cling to the dominant figure in their lives (the abuser) to keep them safe (even though the abuser is the cause of their danger). People who lack the knowledge to get themselves out of danger (especially emotional danger) will often be unable to see a solution, and therefore, lack the imaginative ability (and courage) to move forward. The good news is that imagination can be improved.

How Do You Improve Your Imagination?

If imagination is the key to solving problems and being successful in life, then it is in everyone's interest to improve your imagination. Cherry (2019) quotes psychologist Mihaly Csikszentmihalyi as saying that"of all human activities, creativity comes closest to providing the fulfillment we all hope to get in our lives." This means that imagination (which is perhaps the ultimate expression of creativity) is how we can reach fulfillment in life. Fulfillment is certainly something that we can all hope to have and enjoy.

Operationmeditation.com (n.d.) recommends increasing your imagination as it will open up possibilities for development and change, while Harmer (n.d.)[18] calls imagination a "goal-accomplishing powerhouse." This

---

[18]Harmer, S. (n.d.). 10 Ways to Boost Your Imagination and Achieve Big Things.

already starts to give us a few clues about how to nurture our imagination-through the setting of goals and openness to possibilities. Imagination results in creativity and a sense of accomplishment that comes from seeing our goals reached. However, imagination and creativity are not the same, though they do seem to walk hand in hand. Where imagination is the "fantasy" (or a random combination of associations that we have in our subconscious mind), creativity can be better understood to be the concrete expression of those solutions through their implementation and "creation."

Harmer (n.d.) indicates that stress is detrimental to our imagination. It raises our negativity and makes us feel that we will not reach our goals. It clouds our ability to visualize possibilities. Here are some of the steps that she suggests to boost imagination and reach your potential through creativity:

• **Focus on your potential**

You are what you think (Harmer, n.d.). We need to focus on potential and not challenges. Where your focus is, there your energies will go. Henry Ford, the inventor of the

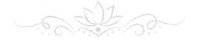

famous American automobile, is famously quoted as saying, "Whether you think you can or you think you can't, you're right." This is really a case of "count your blessings" in a biblical sense. If we focus on all the things we don't have, we will never see what we do have. We certainly won't be able to imagine what we can do with what we do have. In the earlier island scenario, if we focused on the things we don't have (no food, no shelter, no communication, no healthcare, etc.), we would continue to think with a negative mindset. However, if we focused on what we did have (dental floss, a pen, and pantyhose), we can start imagining possibilities that involve what we do have. In this case, the dental floss, pen, and pantyhose were a blessing. Imagination will show us how three random items can keep us fed.

- **Become still**

Harmer (n.d.) also believes in meditation. She writes that in moments when we have inner stillness, such as through meditation, we can begin to disregard the mechanics of logic and open up our subconscious mind, which has infinite possibilities. Hence, it is pretty clear that our logical mind (or conscious mind) can be quite a dampener to the creative processes of the imagination. Instead of thinking about ways that an idea can work, the conscious mind can focus on why it can't or the limitations of why it won't. The subconscious mind and its imagination are unlimited, and if approached in the right manner, we can channel incredible ideas from it. However, first, you need to still your conscious mind or at least teach it to wait before shooting down all your dreams.

• **Redefine you**

We often hear stories about people who ended up in dire straits, with often life-threatening consequences. Sometimes these people manage to go beyond what they thought themselves capable of in order to survive. Aron Ralston has achieved fame with his self-sacrificing (in the literal sense) ordeal when he was trapped by a boulder while rock-climbing. His hand was trapped beneath the massive rock, and he had two choices: wait for help (and possibly die there) or cut off his hand (and possibly die of blood loss, but there's a chance he could hike out and find help). Ralston famously chose the second option (at the end, amputating a part of his arm instead), and he survived. If he had been asked the morning before his climbing expedition if he could cut off his limb, Ralston would have said "no!", and yet when push came to shove, he did just that.

The point is that we often believe that we are defined by our limitations, but this is not necessarily how it should be. Limitations are opportunities for growth and self-exploration. Only in redefining yourself can you realize your full potential and open the doors of creativity. Limitations are stereotypes that need to be broken. Are these some of your limitations?

Limitation	Challenge
I am a girl, I can't change a tire.	Have you tried? It's a skill to learn, not a biologically defined task.
I am not fit enough to participate in the Boston marathon.	People are not born fit, but if you start running just a few miles a day, you may find you like it.
I'm a guy, I can't take up knitting; what will people think?	Many designers are male. You may enjoy expressing your creativity much more than dancing to the beat of someone else's drum.

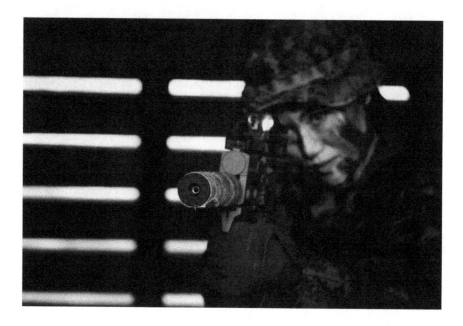

(Image 3.6)

People who are creative and imaginative enjoy challenging their own self-view by doing activities that are out of character. This is a way to test yourself and find out what you are made of. (Image 3.6)

Research

You don't know what you don't know. Let that sink into your conscious mind for a moment. Do you know what it means? It's about knowing. Unless you are God or a higher power, you are not omnipotent, and there is still such an incredible lot out there that you know nothing about.

Hence, it is so frustrating when people (usually teenagers) say "I'm bored." How can anyone ever be bored? There is so much out there to learn, and with the internet, it has become so incredibly easy to do so. Learning new things (especially new skills) is incredibly stimulating for your imagination and your sense of accomplishment. As an example, there was a lady who realized her car's air-filter was blocked, yet the mechanics always neglected to replace it, and as a result, she had to survive the heat in her car with an aircon that didn't work effectively. Welcome to YouTube. After a five-minute tutorial video, she was able to see exactly where the glove-box opened and how to change out the filter herself. It sounds like a silly thing, but this was the moment when she became interested. Once we are "interested," we activate the full power of our minds, and we can achieve things that we never thought were possible. If this seems daunting to you, then remember that researching a task is the best way to "stand on the shoulders of giants" and reach those small goals that lead to your self-development.

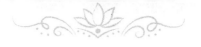

Push, push, push

No, no one is in labor. This is not a Lamaze class, yet it is also exactly what creativity and imagination are like. You are giving birth to your idea. And like real labor, it can be a painful process. Fear, doubts, feelings of inadequacy, and a million other obstacles that try to hold you back will arise and block your way like those contractions that make most women want to have an epidural. In terms of our imagination, there are no short-cuts, though. You have to push, push, push! Hold back your self-judgment and your self-criticism, and, instead, focus on just letting that creative idea be born.

If someone were to criticize your human baby, you would surely protect them with claws, fangs, and lawyers barred? So, why, when it's our imagination's baby, do we just allow others to say things like, "Oh, that's so stupid," "It'll never amount to much," and "Why have you wasted your time on that?" We should defend our imagination (and sometimes, that means defending it from your own inner-critic, too).

The Power of Visualization

Once you start feeling comfortable with embracing your own imagination and the unusual processes that you follow to create an idea, you can begin to use the power of visualization. This is not some magic trick, but rather it is an adaptive skill, meaning that the more we do something, the better we get at it. No, you will probably not be a visualization guru the first time that you try to practice visualization, but with perseverance and by growing your knowledge base of visualization skills, you will achieve all of your goals and lead a more fulfilling life.

Sasson (n.d.) believes that we can use visualization to train our brains to use the power of imaginative thought to realize our goals. If you are not sure what visualization looks like, try the following test:

You are driving along in your car. It is cold and rainy, and the roads are slick, so you are not speeding. The radio station is picking up static, and you glance down to quickly change channels. When you look up, there is a dog in the road ahead of you. You slam on the breaks, and the car slides slightly sideways. Luckily, the dog quickly runs out of the road, and you look at it in the rearview mirror as you drive on.

While reading the above scenario, you might have "seen" the events in your "mind's eye," and you may even have felt your toes tighten in your shoes as you stepped on the brakes as the car was about to hit the dog. Some very creative people even raise their heads slightly to the right (the position of the rearview mirror in the US) to catch a glimpse of the imaginary dog. This is exactly what a visualization looks and feels like. It combines the power of your subconscious mind (through imagination), and it creates a scenario that you can "see" in your mind. This scenario, obviously, doesn't have to be traumatic, like this one, and it can serve as a way to prepare for life-changes.

Consider the following developmental visualization that you may consider using before an important job interview: (note that it is in the present tense and uses the first-person).

I am driving my car on my way to the new company where I hope to work. The day is clear, and I can see for miles off to the left where the coast stretches into the sea. The smell of salty tang on the air is refreshing. Pulling into the parking lot at JB

Enterprises, I find a visitor's parking space in the shade and step out of the car, pausing on the passenger's side to collect my resume and notepad for the job interview. Walking up to the entrance, I smile as the impressive glass doors slide open to admit me into the glossy oak veneer offices. The receptionist is friendly, and she asks me to wait just a minute while she checks if the managers are available.

I barely sit on the classy suede seat when she comes around the counter to lead me to the conference room. She politely holds the door open for me, and I step inside to meet with the three managers, who are responsible for the filling of vacancies.

This visualization contains several positive elements to form an attachment to the beautiful surroundings, the pleasure of being near the beach, the anticipated rewards from landing the job, and the sense of confidence that they develop through the creative visualization process. The more details you can add to the visualization, the better the image builds in your minds. It is like laying a path before your feet to follow quite easily through the problems in your life.

Sports players also rehearse before they go out on the field for the final game. All those training matches ensure that the team is where it needs to be when it needs to be there. Likewise, visualization is a way for you to practice events like job interviews, saying your marriage vows, and even going to the bank for a loan application and in this way make those events less terrifying. But it can also be used to "see" the solutions to problems. Inventors usually "see" their invention long before it appears on paper or as a finished model.

Visualization can also be something that is shared. At companies, they often talk about a shared vision or a belief of where their company is heading. Our visualizations can be driven by events around us, and this can also become a scary and even dangerous situation for us. Remember, the subconscious mind is the survival brain. It will use any tool at its disposal to prepare the body for fight or flight to survive at any cost. There have been documented cases of mass-hysteria all across the world where people had such a strong shared belief that their visualizations also became similar. (Like seeing aliens in New Mexico in the 1950s.) We often see this in incidences where there have been an outbreak of a disease or contagious disease. Suddenly, everyone has symptoms! (Or at least, think that they do.) Social media has become the latest platform for spreading large-scale visualizations and encouraging people to panic. Sadly, this is not what visualization is meant to do. There are numerous studies into the effectiveness of visualization to conquer our fears, reach achievements, develop skills, and guide the process of mental transformations.

Studies to Back up the Effectiveness of Visualization

Whenever a "new" psychological method takes off (especially when it gets snapped up by thousands of online wanna-be gurus), it is often subject to intense scrutiny from the elite circles in the psychology and medical fields. Even psychoanalysis (which is now an established field of study) had similar struggles in its infancy. People tend to criticize when they see something new taking off even if that something is not so new. Currently, the debate about the medicinal consumption of cannabis oil and other such products is raging through the same circles, with many acting as strong proponents, while there is also massive opposition. The same is also happening to the concept of visualization as a means for boosting our confidence, dealing with mental concepts, and harmful constructs (beliefs). The world is shouting about visualization on the internet, and though some people will be quick to judge and label something as being "snake-oil," there are still millions of people worldwide who firmly believe in the power of visualization and meditation.

Adams (2009)[19] believes that visualization is, in essence, "mental practice," where we go through a scene that we believe will happen in the near future (whether it is a desire of ours or an imminent reality). According to research, referenced by Adams (2009), when we think of the activity, it is almost as good as doing that activity, though, practicing both the thinking and the doing will yield even better results. What this means for visualization believers is

---

[19]Adams, A.J. (2009). Seeing Is Believing: The Power of Visualization: Your best life, from the comfort of your armchair.

that we can indeed accomplish much with visualization (mental practice), but it still works even better when we get off our bums and we get physically cracking at the idea or task. If you want to become a talented writer, it means that, though it helps to dream or visualize yourself accepting a Pulitzer prize, it is still going to be necessary for you to pick up a pen and write 'till your fingers bleed.

In a well-documented study by Guang Yue, a psychologist specializing in exercise at the Cleveland Clinic Foundation in Ohio, people who attended gym were compared with those who didn't. The difference being that those who didn't go for regular exercise routines were taught about visualization, and they would spend as much time every day at home (in their armchairs) mentally doing the exercises. In other words, they would visualize themselves doing push-ups, lunges, and running on the treadmill. After the tests were completed, the group who physically went to the gym to do the activities had gained 30% muscle mass. However, the test subjects who had done only the visualization had also picked up muscle mass (without lifting a finger)! Their muscle mass increased by 13.5%. Both groups of subjects retained this effect for up to three months after the tests were concluded. This proves that even thinking about something can create a physical change (Adams, 2009). If visualization was not able to deliver what it promised, then it would certainly not be so popular among a wealth of public figures, who all admit to using visualization to improve their careers and lives.

Williams (n.d.)[20] refers to several prominent public figures such as Jim Carrey, Arnold Schwarzenegger, and Oprah Winfrey who use visualization to reach their goals. Each of these people has set and reached their goals through visualization. What is exceptionally interesting is that each of these individuals found their own way to take their visualizations and make them into something concrete -a way to commit to the goals that their dreams had set.

Jim Carrey

The comedian/actor is a huge fan and promoter of visualization and the concept of the Law of Attraction (where you essentially believe that the universe has

---

[20] Williams, A. (n.d.). 8 Successful People Who Use The Power Of Visualization.

everything you need, and your attitude and mental preparedness will attract all that you need to you), and he shared some of his top tips with Daniels (n.d.). He states that "you can't just visualize and go eat a sandwich." Elaborating on this, he states that you have to see where you want to go and put in the action to get there. Hence, you can visualize, but you need to do the work (sorry, visualizing that you will win the lottery is not going to improve your wealth).

Carrey also believes that our lives are a result of our intentions and desires. What you want to do (if you want it badly enough) will drive your life towards that purpose. He believed this so sincerely that in 1990 Carrey wrote himself a "paycheck" for 10 million dollars but he dated it for 1994. Four years later (in 1994), Carrey landed his first huge acting role where he earned (you guessed it) 10 million dollars. Jim Carrey is an example of belief in action. He visualized his goals and made the first commitment to it by writing himself a check (four years in advance) to symbolize his vision.

Arnold Schwarzenegger

The huge *Terminator* action hero and statesman, who has been an inspiration to millions of fans worldwide, is also a huge fan of visualization. His rags-to-riches story is one based on visualization. According to Robertson (2015), Schwarzenegger's visualizations started as a young boy when he saw a poster of Reg Park, the star of the movie *Hercules*, and this inspired the young boy to become a bodybuilder. Schwarzenegger saw an image (a visual) of what he wanted to be and he began to plan for that dream (with visualization). Robertson (2015)[21] explains this by saying that Schwarzenegger used visualization, which preceded the accomplishment of his goals. However, vision starts with an inspiration, and before you can visualize, you need to be interested enough to believe.

Schwarzenegger's rise to fame in the bodybuilding ranks and the world of Hollywood is also greatly attributed to his dedication, effort, and hard work. Muscles don't build themselves to look like Schwarzenegger. It requires continued effort. If not for that, we may never have heard of

---

[21]Robertson, C. (2015). How Arnold Schwarzenegger Used a Vision To Achieve Greatness - And You Can Too.

the young boy from the Austrian village. He would still have sat dreaming with his *Hercules* poster if he had not put in the effort to develop his visualizations.

Oprah Winfrey

Although we know Ms. Winfrey as a TV talk show host and public figure, she had always dreamed of being an actress. Achelles (2018)[22] writes that the woman we all know as Oprah had dreamed of the role in *The Color Purple* for months in advance. She envisioned herself reading the lines, filming the role, and achieving her dream – of being an actress. Oprah is also a huge subscriber of the beliefs of the Law of Attraction. She believes that in imagining ourselves doing what we want or dream of (visualization), we can align the energies (or perhaps it's really the subconscious mind?), and achieve our goals (because we have created communication between the conscious mind or desire and the subconscious mind or imagination and, therefore, achieved our goals).

---

[22]Achelles, R. (2018). Oprah Winfrey credits her success to this one thing we all have.

How Science Uses Visualization

From these famous people's experiences with visualization, it is clear that visualization is real. But making our visions real is up to us. With the development of science, we have been able to test exactly how powerful visualization is. Matthew Nagle, a C4 quadriplegic, received a ground-breaking procedure where an interface between his mind and a computer was designed and surgically implanted for him. This exciting procedure has resulted in Nagle being able to control a cursor on the computer screen, move a robot arm around, and even play games. How does he do it? Through visualization. He uses his brain (specifically his conscious and subconscious mind) to achieve what able-bodied people do every day. The mobility of his body has been taken over by various machines and technologies; however, his mind is still exactly what we all have – a brain with a conscious and subconscious mind. His brain is capable of visualization, and Nagel is achieving his goals in measurable terms (Martin, 2005)[23].

---

[23]Martin, R. (2005). Mind Control.

With influential (and successful) people and highly scientific studies such as that by Guang Yue proving that visualization is real and it has the power to change your life by setting your goals and helping you practice how to reach those goals, isn't it time to become a believer in visualization?

How to Make Practical Use of Imagination

Okay, so you're still on the fence on the whole visualization-use-your-imagination hype, but you're willing to give it a bash – here's how. To be practically successful at recharging your imagination (let's be honest, your imagination switched off when you turned all serious and adult-like), you need to awaken the inner child (your subconscious mind) and get curious about the world around you again. If you are faced with a huge challenge and have just read somewhere that imagination is great for solving challenges, don't suddenly expect to close your eyes and – Wham! – you're a genius. Problem solved.

Imagination involves the brain, and like studying for exams, it requires practice and repetition.

When you learned about mathematics for the first time, your teacher didn't throw Calculus at you in grade school. You started with baby steps (one plus one), and this is the same approach to take in awakening your imagination. You need to develop a partnership with your mind and build up those mental muscles, so when you do need them in a few weeks down the line, they are bulging and ready to deliver.

- **Get curious**

As we explained in Part One of this book, our subconscious mind creates routines because they are safe and they keep everything in life ticking along "nice and smooth." Unfortunately, routines are also very effective at killing our imaginations. To develop curiosity, you need to do something other than what you have always done, anything else except what you know and trust is a good start. It doesn't have to be huge decisions, and the goal is not to reinvent yourself (though you may end up doing that anyway). The goal is just to start thinking about your life and your decisions again and to get out of the mental rut that you are in.

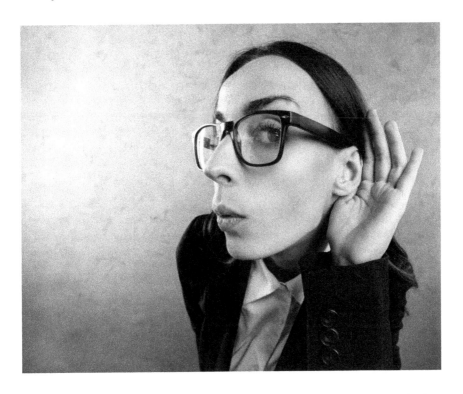

Curiosity is about how we see the world. Find a new and exciting way to look at the ordinary. There doesn't have to be a reason for it, except to try something different and "see what if…" (Image 3.7)

John F Kennedy, U.S President and world-famous leader, is quoted as saying, "Change is the law of life. And those who look only to the past or present are certain to miss the future." Change is often scary, but only by changing our mindset and approaching new situations and new choices with a spirit of curiosity can we rewire the brain. Kennedy may not have known about visualization in his era as we know about it today, but he understood that our future depends on what we do today. If we keep on doing what we've always been doing, nothing will change. Consider the following questions concerning your life; where could you begin to explore and imagine alternatives? (Where could you make a change?)

When you buy groceries, do you buy the same product every time? Have you considered trying a new product or shopping at a new store entirely? (And this is about more than just where there are bargains.)

If you were driving a pick-up for the last two years and it's time for a trade-in, do you immediately consider another pick-up? Would you consider buying an SUV or even a motorcycle? (There are always practical issues to consider, yet most of us will not even go test-drive a different type or brand of vehicle to what we already have.)

Do you always take the same route to work in the morning? Perhaps you can take a different route or stop at a different coffee shop? (Do you even see the landscape or scenery that is along your old route?)

When last did you browse something different on the internet or Facebook? If you are a business owner, perhaps look into the outdoors or recycling initiatives. Find something new to be interested in again.

When last did you write something by hand? We live in a digital era with apps and programs for every possible form of note-taking. Yet, psychologists will agree, there is something about writing by hand that activates the brain in a way so different from typing.

This list of questions could be unending, but all of it boils down to questioning what you take for granted or what your brain has made into a routine. If you think of a five-year-old child, they are always questioning their world, which is normal since it is how they learn. As adults, we tend to stop learning about our worlds, and once we start questioning our worlds and use words like "Why? How come? Does it...?" we will begin to evaluate our life decisions and set new goals. We will begin to imagine again.

Go somewhere new

This is not a vacation. It doesn't have to be a trip to Paris or Bali. Just go somewhere new, spend some time in a new venue, and open your eyes to this new world. If you spend your whole day in the office, perhaps go sit at a local market and watch the people and the routines they have. As they carry on with their business, allow your mind to take note of the ways in which they have dealt with challenges. This is an activity of seeing how others use imagination to improve their lives. At the end of the day, begin to look at the challenges (goals) in your life and start to wonder how you can solve those goals.

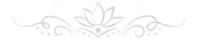

Give yourself time

Whenever we have a moment to ourselves, isn't it strange how we end up spending it on something other than ourselves? When we have a minute in the line at the grocery store, we are checking our emails. At the end of the day, we spend time "catching up" on social media instead of catching up on "us." Yet, we always complain that we don't have time to visualize, we don't have time to meditate, and we don't have time to change. Avoiding technology is a great way to find the time. It may only be a few minutes at first, but once you claim those precious minutes and assign it to your imagination, you will begin to imagine having a little bit more time for, let's say, meditation. With focus, you will put in the work to please your imagination and make more time. Each time you can find even a few minutes to invest in yourself, you will see a goal ticked off on your list. Creative people, who reach their goals, who embrace and create opportunities, are not lucky. That type of "luck is preparation meeting opportunity" (Oprah Winfrey, n.d.). Our imagination can create opportunities if we let it by giving ourselves time.

Imagine your goals

When we have a goal to reach or the result of a challenge to achieve, we are giving our subconscious mind the information to create a plan of action in our mind with our imagination. According to PracticalLifeReflection.com (n.d.), we have to imagine our goals, visualize them in complete detail, and then we will begin moving towards achievement. So, when you are taking the train home after work and your goal is to one day own your first car, you can begin to visualize sitting behind the wheel of that car. Looking out the window of the train, you can "see" yourself driving home with a happy smile on your face as you shift gears or turn at intersections. Move your feet as you imagine yourself stepping on the gas pedal or feel the grip of the steering wheel in your hands. Eventually, that visualization will grow as your imagination expands. You might see a briefcase on the seat next to you in the car and realize that you want to change your job too. It might inspire you to go to night school to finish your diploma and, thereby, allow you to apply to another company or even change careers entirely - all because you had a vision of you driving your first car.

Imagine your goals again, and again

Seeing yourself driving that car is not good enough if you only do it once. Your imagination will not keep planning if you don't keep laying down the mental tracks for its journey. You need to visualize daily. Whenever you have a spare moment, see your goal, imagine the steps to reach it. You can even begin to write down the steps to reaching that goal that your imagination has laid out for you. Remember, Jim Carrey wrote himself a check for 10 million dollars, but he also had a date in mind, and he worked tirelessly to reach that "deadline." You can too.

Imagination works when we do. It is not just about having your head up in the clouds or dreaming up wonderful lives, which we secretly believe we will never have. It is actionable planning, free from the pessimism that our conscious mind (based upon the negative memories and experiences stored in the subconscious mind) has accepted as our daily routines. With these practical applications of imagination mentioned here, you can begin to nourish your starving imagination and conceive of a better life for yourself, plan the goals to reach your new reality, and work out a roadmap of how to get there. Your imagination can be the GPS to guide you on an exciting new life journey if you give yourself the time to dream and take the actions to make those dreams a reality.

Auto-Suggestion: The Medium for Influencing the Subconscious Mind

Auto-suggestion is a greatly misunderstood concept in creating change in our lives. It is not brainwashing, though it may seem like it. Worstell (2019)[24] explains that auto-suggestion refers to all the stimuli we can intentionally send into our subconscious mind and that this needs to be intentionally administered through our senses such as taste, touch, hearing, seeing, and speaking. This means that it is the influx of information that originates with our intentions into our brains. When you tell yourself that you are beautiful, it is an auto-suggestion. The "suggestion" part comes into play because we can't make our minds

---

[24]Worstell, R.C. (2019). Auto-suggestion – Influencing the Subconscious Mind.

believe something. We can only suggest it. The more we suggest it, the better the chances that our brain will accept it to be true and, therefore, believe it.

You might consider it to be like wanting your mind to dance to a particular song. If you only play the first beat, you will not get much of a response, but if you play all of the beats, it will create the rhythm, and soon your mental feet will be tapping along. Therefore, for auto-suggestion to be effective, we need to repeat it over a lengthy period of time. How long will depend on what you are trying to achieve (your goal). If it is something like wanting to learn to swim, and you've never had the chance before, it will be a reasonably easy thing to do. You could watch movies with scenes of swimming, place pictures of people swimming in the ocean all around your work station, and even listen to the sounds of the ocean on your iPod. This will all increase your desire to learn how to swim, and if you added the visualizing of yourself swimming happily in a dam or pool, you would soon be on your way to getting your toes wet.

However, if you wanted to learn to swim, but you had a traumatic event happen to you previously such as drowning, it will be a lot more difficult to achieve this goal.

Your auto-suggestions will need to be much stronger since they need to create a new thinking paradigm while breaking down the old structure that your subconscious mind had created. Your subconscious mind is there to preserve your life. If you had suffered a near-death experience due to almost drowning, it will definitely fight you (guns blazing) with negative thoughts if you suddenly want to learn how to swim. You will need to reprogram your subconscious mind if you wish to make swimming a goal and hope to achieve it. Remember, your subconscious mind will be soaked in the emotions that went with your past experience. It will quickly remind you of almost choking on the water, the fear, and helplessness. You will need to convince it that learning to swim has more benefits than a few bad memories and that it is really quite safe.

There are a few ways to reach the subconscious mind. If you recall, we have already explained in Part One that the subconscious mind is not in direct contact with our conscious mind where our desires originate. We need to get the information to it in a round-about way. The "subconscious mind resembles a fertile garden spot, in which weeds will grow in abundance if the seeds of more desirable crops are not sown therein" (Worstell, 2019). You need to "seed" your subconscious with a "desirable crop."

To get our information or "seeds" across to the subconscious mind, we can use the following ways:

Theta brain waves

When the brain is in theta state (just before we go to sleep or wake up), the conscious mind has begun to let go of its control mechanisms (like evaluating things, thinking, planning, and remembering what happened today). At the same time, the subconscious mind starts to check its information highways, and it becomes much more alert to the information, which the mind receives from the senses (sound, touch/vibration, smell, and to a lesser extent, taste). The subconscious mind is now open to our suggestions in the form of stimuli.

Sounds or words introduced during theta brainwave states will be directly admitted into the subconscious mind. However, it is not a one-time-only offer. This is like a marriage – you're in it for the long haul. You need to show

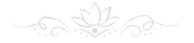

up daily and keep repeating what you want to change. It's like every time you input new information, you are laying a brick to climb over a wall. Except, this is the Great Wall of China, so you will need a lot of bricks! In psychological terms, when we want to change habitual behavior, such as being scared of swimming and water or being an alcoholic, we need to change the information for 21-28 days to get across the highway of behavior. (This is why rehab centers tend to keep their clients for a period of 28-30 days.)

So, if you want to convince your subconscious mind that you can and should go learn to swim, you might start with affirmations spoken during the presence of theta brainwaves. Since you will be half asleep at this point, it will be necessary for you to record your affirmations or even purchase a suitable system that does this. Some companies can create your own affirmation recording with a voice and backing music that falls within the correct decibel range and at the correct frequency to further enhance your experience and results. Your affirmations might be something like:

I am happy in the water.

There is peace in the water.

I feel the water flow over my body and I swim with grace.

There is nothing to fear in the water.

I am safe as I learn to swim.

My body is strong and will keep me safe while I swim.

I am stronger than my past, and I can rewrite what happened.

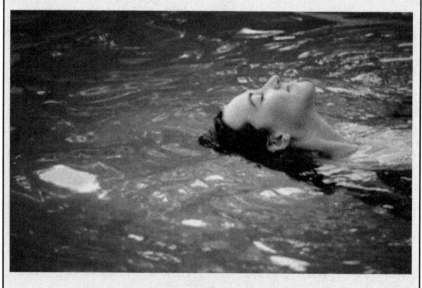

(Image 3.8)

Visualization

Using our eyes, with sight being one of our strongest

senses, we can further program the subconscious mind by

using auto-suggestion. Putting up images of the ocean, swimming, and playing in the waves all contribute to experiences that can fuel our imagination. We can strengthen this by clearing our mind (through meditation) of negative thoughts and memories that the subconscious mind uses to maintain its current routines (such as a fear of drowning and remembering how it felt when the water closed over your head when you almost drowned in the past). Once you feel a sense of peace, your brain waves will also slow down, reaching beta and alpha (the states just above theta) where your worries decrease, allowing for the subconscious mind to actually pay attention to our imagination. At this point, you can begin visualizing positive thoughts (about the desired outcome) of learning to swim.

You could see yourself lying in shallow water at first, splashing happily, and perhaps even floating lightly on the waves. Your mind moves from the known to the unknown, which is how it learns, so it's best not to overwhelm it initially. Visualizing yourself diving head-first into a pool will only scare your subconscious mind and make that Great Wall even higher.

Once you can happily see yourself playing in the shallows and feeling content, you can slowly progress to deeper water. Distractions such as details of the beautiful creatures in the water or the presence of your swimming instructor nearby to keep you safe can also help your subconscious mind to swallow the thought of learning to swim easier.

Visualization needs to be (you guessed it) repeated.

Repetitions

When you were a child at school, you learned how to do things by repeating them. If you can recall, learning your ABCs wasn't done in only a day. It took the better part of your first school year. You sang the ABC song, you wrote out the letters, and drew pictures for each letter. All of this was different forms of repetition. Like forming a footpath through the wilds, if you walk on the same patch of land over and over again, you will make a path. And the next time that you walk there, the going will be just a little bit easier.

The same holds true for your mind. If you can get the same information into the subconscious mind over and over again, you add bricks to your new superhighway that will cancel out the old Great Wall. So, while you are in the theta state, you repeat affirmations and you calm your mind with meditation and then repeat the visualizations, all the while, forming that new footpath through the wilds of your mind.

Worstell (2019) states that the lack of repetition is the number one reason why people get no change in their lives despite "trying" visualization and affirmations. The problem is that you can't simply "try" it. You have to commit to it, and you have to commit to it long term. If you have been struggling with negative thoughts for most of your adult life, and you decide that you want to be positive from now on, you can't simply change your behavior on one rainy Saturday afternoon and expect lasting change to occur.

Influencing the subconscious mind is a lengthy process, but it is such a vital process since our negative behaviors affect not only ourselves but also the people around us. *SpiritualResearchFoundation.org* (n.d.) finds that our

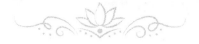

negative behaviors become personality defects. Like an amputee, the person who is displaying the negative behavior is lacking something. Their acting out or entrenched behaviors are like phantom limb syndrome, and even though the original cause of their behavior is now gone, they still keep following the same behavior patterns. Auto-suggestions are a means of re-attaching the severed limb, but it will take a while to heal.

The repetition of the auto-suggestions is so important because, like that newly attached limb, there may be setbacks that can compromise the healing. The limb may develop an infection, for instance, and likewise, your visualizations may be dealt a blow when you have a panic attack the first time you set foot in the shallows at the beach. The important thing is not to throw in the towel. Don't simply stop because it gets hard or difficult. Keep going, keep up with the repetitions, and soon you will have created the new neural pathways that will support your desires and help you reach your goals.

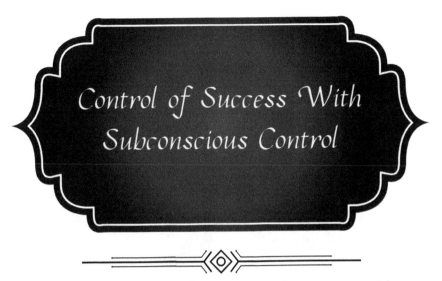

Control of Success With Subconscious Control

Before we can seek to control success with our subconscious mind, we need to explore and decide what success means to us. Success does not mean the same thing to everyone. This is perhaps why so many people reach the goals that they have set, yet they do not feel that it is enough and feel unsatisfied. Jasin (2017)[25] explores success and finds that sometimes we rely on others to tell us what success is because we don't really know what it is ourselves. We strive for something that was never even important to us in the first place. When you accept someone else's version of what success looks like, you will

---

[25]Jasin, A. (2017). What Does Success Really Mean to You?

feel a definite let down once you reach what you thought was your "goal."

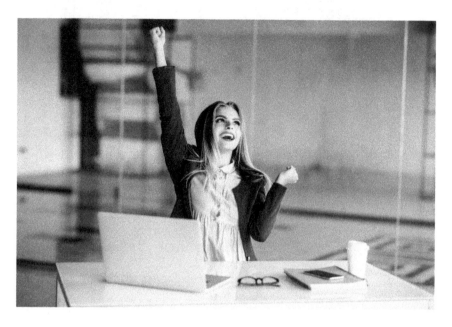

(Image 4.1)

It is very easy to listen to what society tells us our goals should be. Success will only matter to us when it is the attainment of something that makes us feel content and satisfied. There is no need to apologize for what makes you happy; it is your decision. (Image 4.1)

Jacob (2019)[26] creates a unique set of views on success by interviewing several highly successful people to find out what their definitions of success are. She quotes Paige Arnof-Fenn, CEO of Mavens & Moguls, who says that

---

[26] Jacob, C. (2019). What Is Success? (Great Answers from 35 Successful People).

"success is very personal so your definition will be - and should be - different than mine." This reiterates the view that success is not a generic term. Other successful business leaders added their voices in saying that real success comes not from reaching the finish line only, and that the efforts and experiences of the race to that success is equally important. Life is about the journey and not the destination; you should enjoy the scenery along the way, since you spend more time on the journey than the destination in any case.

Interestingly enough, most of these really successful (and wealthy) people do not list money or status as being integral to being successful. It seems that the old adage holds true, "money can't buy you happiness." Social media fuels the belief that success means money, fame, and wealth. It pollutes our senses with images of pricey clothes, lifestyles, and values that might, in the end, not make you happy at all (Jasin, 2017).

Key points reached by top achievers have been identified by Jacob (2019):

- Moving forward
- True to yourself

- Achieving your goals

- Find meaning in your work

- Experiencing the life journey

- You design success for yourself, and the definition is allowed to change

- Live on your own terms

- A life of integrity and perseverance

To reach these key points, it is essential that you discover and develop control, confidence, willpower, and focus, as well as a determination to reach goals. Only then will you be able to claim and prove to yourself that you are successful, at which point, the opinions of other people will no longer matter, and happiness will follow.

Take Control of Your Life

Dr. Phil McGraw (2002, p. 225),[27] international psychologist and TV personality, explains that we all have a "pattern of response, unique to [us], [and this] is a characteristic that is called your locus of control." This

---

[27] McGraw, P. (2002). Self Matters: Creating Your Life From The Inside Out. Pocket Books: Berkshire.

means that each of us has a place where we believe the control of our lives is found. Those who believe that they have an internal locus of control place responsibility for their lives at their own feet. They believe that they create their lives and that they have the power to take action to change what happens to them. As McGraw writes, it tells us where we think the responsibility for our lives lie and who or what is to blame for the events in your life.

Your subconscious mind also has a say in where your locus of control lies. It is not something that you get to simply decide on. It is like the traffic controller in your subconscious mind. It will integrate information that supports its view of who is responsible for your life into your subconscious mind based upon your pre-existing thinking patterns. Caprino (2015)[28] believes that only with a mindshift can people take control of their lives, and only when people see things in a different light or perspective, can we act in a new and liberating way. She also continues to urge that people take action to reclaim their lives and control, and that even small actions can make a difference in who you see as being in control of your life.

---

[28]Caprino, C. (2015). Six Ways To Take Back Control Of Your Life.

Caprino also refers to the ever popular *Chicken Soup for the Soul* series and shares some of the tips from a book in the series that is all about reclaiming your life.

Me time

When we budget our time, we tend to hand it out to others, things, and events. How often do we budget time for ourselves? It is about claiming a part of your time for yourself, to do whatever you want to do for you. This is important since it establishes yourself as an important person in your own life. Too often, we tend to place our needs and wants on the back-burner of life. If we don't value ourselves, and we don't see ourselves as important, why should others do so?

Break stereotypes

We are often held in place by the dictates of society. Our minds, with convictions placed on us by our peers, our culture, and our societies, tell us constantly that we can't do certain things. Taking control of our lives is about doing just that. You step up and launch yourself out of the chains of stereotypical thinking.

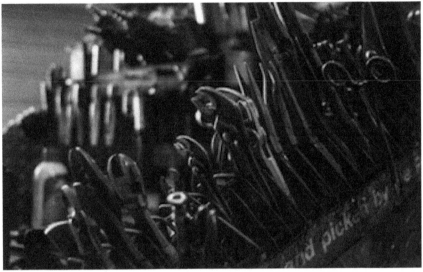

(Image 4.2)

Taking control means "being" the right tool for your job and not letting others tell you that you're not. (Image 4.2)

Respect

We tend to give respect to our peers, our bosses, and our colleagues, yet we often neglect giving respect to ourselves. There is a constant stream of information (a conversation if you like) between your conscious mind and your subconscious mind. This is the way in which you talk to, with, and about yourself. If you don't treat yourself with respect, it will have harmful consequences in life. People with good self-esteem tend to treat themselves as they treat others. Even the Bible talks of this when it says "love thy neighbor as you love yourself." The problem is that many people don't love themselves, and they can't, therefore, love their neighbors. This love starts from our formative years where we learned to respect others and also ourselves. You can check on your self-respect levels by monitoring the inner monologue that your mind has with you, or, as some call it, your self-talk. Do you say the following?

Examples of negative self-talk, which indicates a low self-respect and low self-esteem.	"You fool, why did you do that?" "I knew I shouldn't have tried that." "What will people think?" "No one will believe you." "See, you're on your own again." "I'm not good enough." "I don't trust myself."
Examples of positive or neutral self-talk, which indicates a high level of self-respect and high self-esteem.	"I can do better next time." "I tried, and I learned a valuable lesson." "I think..." "I believe in myself." "I have nothing to prove." "I am good; I am enough." "I can trust myself; I have a proven track record."

People who engage in negative self-talk have no self-respect and tend to blame the world for their woes. Those with positive self-talk usually have an internal locus of control and see the world as a place with opportunities where they can prove themselves to themselves. They take control by setting goals and achieving those goals.

The Confidence That Comes With Control

One of the hardest skills to learn is saying "no." We are pressured into always giving in, always copping out when we really don't want to do something. Secretly, we believe that if we say "no," people will cease to like or approve of us. It is, therefore, an indicator of a low self-esteem and an external locus of control. People in this state are incapable of saying "no" since they lack the power to do so. They lack confidence in their own abilities and especially in their ability to say "no" and live with the consequences of this decision.

Once you master the skill of saying "no" and not caving in when the person you've turned down applies pressure, you will begin to feel a sense of confidence. It is a trust in your own decision making skills and in the validity of your judgments. Many of us get bullied into agreeing to things that we really don't want to do, buy, or be a part of. This is disempowering, and if allowed to continue, boosts the view that you are not in control of your life and that your decisions are made by others. Clearly, this will influence your confidence negatively.

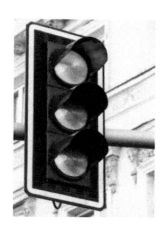

(Image 4.3)

Saying "no" is an important skill that we should practice in life. It is not about being difficult or unhelpful, but it is rather about being in control and being responsible for our actions or the choice not to take action. (Image 4.3)

Taking back your self-confidence is about taking control. But if you have already lost control, you need to start at the very beginning. Your first steps.

If you could remember that far back (most of us can't), you would remember that your first unassisted baby steps were a pretty big deal. Before those first wobbly steps, you were reliant on others to get around, and if no one was around to help, you had to crawl to get around.

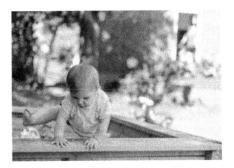

(Image 4.4)

Our baby steps are the first challenges of independence in life. When we succeed, we develop confidence because we have taken control. (Image 4.4)

When you were helped up before you felt ready, you would cry. If you fell down, you would cry. But you didn't give up. It was a struggle (thank goodness for that diaper that absorbed most of the hard landings), but it was also a process of try, fail, try again. It was your first lesson in life, and it was about not giving up, not letting others be responsible for your progress, and the sense of achievement that came when you successfully walked those first few steps without your terrified parents watching. That achievement, and all the achievements since (running, climbing, riding a bicycle, and tying shoe laces) have contributed to building confidence.

So, to rebuild your shattered confidence (life can be pretty rough and damaging to our self-esteem and our confidence levels then plummet) you need to give yourself baby steps to show and convince your subconscious mind that you can be trusted and you can succeed. The best way to do this is with micro-tasks. Doing something new in life (since your subconscious mind is already convinced that you suck at those things you do know) will give you an opportunity to achieve small successes.

You could take up a new sport, a new hobby, start studying a short course, or travel to a new place (even if it's just a new coffee shop you've been meaning to check out). These new experiences will all come with their own information and opportunities to take action. If you have lost your control over yourself, you have lost the ability to make decisions and move forward (you probably tend to wonder what someone else would do in a situation), and if you force yourself to move forward, you encourage yourself to do things, be things, and act instead of reacting.

According to Markway (2018)[29] control (and the confidence that comes with it) can be seen in almost all happy and successful people. Without self-confidence we will be afraid (like the baby that falls before succeeding at the first steps). Markway also believes that with an increased self-confidence we can silence the negative self-talk and take even more control over our lives. Quy (2016)[30] expands on this in saying that most leaders are known for the confidence that they have not only in themselves but also in the confidence that they instill in their subordinates. Whenever we think of who is in control, we think of the boss, the proverbial leader. It is their responsibility to step up and make decisions. This requires confidence. Without confidence, there is no leadership and no control.

Great leaders are often said to have a vision, and they are excellent at getting people to act in line with their vision. When President Franklin Roosevelt was elected after the Great Depression, he had to use his abilities to control, inspire, and motivate people into participating in his public

[29]Markway, B. (2018). Why Self-Confidence Is More Important Than You Think.

[30]Quy, L. (2016). 7 Mental Hacks to Be More Confident in Yourself.

works projects. The American people believed him because he had confidence. Great leaders have confidence because they know that they are in control. They are not waiting for someone else to come and fix the problems that they are in charge of fixing. They have an internal locus of control, they know their skills, and their greatest asset becomes their confidence. Building this confidence also requires willpower and focus to achieve the goals that we set throughout life.

Willpower and Focus

Silvestre (2018)[31] believes that it is a biological urge or characteristic of our DNA code that we seek to improve ourselves. In the wilds, it is really a case of survival of the fittest or most ingenious. As a result of this, we are on a constant quest for self-discovery and self-betterment. In our careers, we want to get a promotion. In our relationships, we want to have children, since we often try

---

[31] Silvestre, D. (2018). 10 Ways to Improve Your Willpower and Regain Your Strength

to "fix our errors" in our children (sort of version 2.0 of our DNA). Even in a spiritual sense, we aim for improvement, to earn our way up to heaven. This quest for betterment and improvement requires that we develop our willpower or personal perseverance.

Working for personal betterment and keeping your willpower charged can be an exhausting process that is ongoing throughout life. This is more than simple physical fatigue but also refers to the mental strain that we suffer as we struggle through life (sort of a mental wear-and-tear of our life engines or drive to success). Changing old habits can be especially hard, and your subconscious mind will fight you all the way since it doesn't like change. At times it may seem that you lack the willpower to move forward and break the negative cycles of your life.

There are a few ways in which to strengthen your willpower according to Silvestre (2018). Some of these ways may seem quite logical, though we tend to neglect them (and ourselves) when it comes to boosting our willpower.

Get enough sleep

Getting enough sleep daily is essential to keeping your body running smoothly. It cuts down on the stress that you suffer when your body enters a state of discomfort from not running properly. With a fresh mind, you will have more go in your life, keep a sense of positivity, and stop your subconscious mind from screaming "attack!

Meditate

Meditation is synonymous with the idea of stillness. When you are driving yourself at 120 miles an hour down the highway of instructions in your mind, it is a good idea to become still every couple of hours. This will cut out fatigue and unnecessary stress.

Good habits

Unfortunately, when we feel we're not coping, we tend to turn to outside "help" in the form of smoking, drinking, and drugs. These do not help you cope better; they are simply distractions from the real issues. Forming good coping habits will help you much more effectively in the long run. Going for a run or listening to soothing music when you are feeling up tight will be a better solution and certainly do less damage than a vice such as smoking will.

Block unnecessary decisions and create focus	There is only so much that you can decide about each day. Use routines to make life a little bit more predictable and cut out thinking (and sweating) the small stuff. Choose what you want to wear the night before work, eat the same breakfast and lunch (then spoil yourself for supper), and keep your office organized the same way, so you don't have to go look for things and waste mental energy.
Chip at the mountain	When we are faced with overwhelming tasks or decisions in life, it is a good idea to look at the foothills and not focus on the summit (which may seem impossible to reach). If you are deciding to change to a different career, you could begin working a few hours a day at the new career while still keeping your old job as a way to test the waters. This would remove a lot of unnecessary stress and keep you motivated.

Focus is the ability to keep your eye on the prize, despite the distractions that may seek to prevent your satisfaction of your goals. For instance, when you hand in your resignation so that you can start a new career, your old boss gives you a better financial offer or a raise in an attempt to keep you from leaving. This was not your goal, as you really want to change careers to something that will be more fulfilling to you. With focus, you will be able to have the willpower to keep going despite the temptation of more money and reach your original goal. If you lack focus, you will easily cave and accept the offer (choosing the known over the unknown).

Your willpower and focus can be depleted; they are not infinite. Temptations, negativity, and physical or mental exhaustion can be detrimental to your progress. Cummins (2013)[32] suggests a few ways to keep focused and energized. She believes that you should ration your willpower use to prevent it being used up, while imagination can certainly be used to keep a calm state of mind and promote relaxation (stress is very bad for our willpower, and it blunts our focus).

Cummins also refers to thought substitution. This is when you train your brain to think of something else when

---

[32]Cummins, D. (2013). How to Boost Your Willpower: Willpower is like a muscle —in more ways than one.

a particular thought comes into your mind. A repetitive thought is how we suffer from cravings (your subconscious mind loves repetitions). So, if you are prone to thinking of failure, you can substitute that thought with an image of a big shiny trophy. Your brain, through repetition, will begin to automatically make the association if you intentionally repeat it enough. Practically, this means that your mind will be less likely to believe you are going to fail if the image of a beautiful trophy appears in your mind's eye at the same time.

With the correct amount of willpower, focus, and the confidence to reach your goals, you will be able to control your life.

Goal Achievement

The achievement of our goals is integral to developing a sense of well-being and accomplishment in life. If we never reach or do what we set out to, this will negatively influence our sense of self-worth, and, over time, it will create a poor self-esteem and external locus of control (we blame everyone but ourselves). In sharp contrast, those who regularly reach their goals (no matter how small those are) will be forward thinking, proud of their achievements, and confident in their ability to do more. These people will have an internal locus of control (they accept responsibility and run with ideas).

Achievement is linked to accomplishing goals. However, often we do not set realistic goals or have our goals dictated to us by others. Reaching these goals will not offer us the satisfaction that we require to build our self-confidence. Goals that are too easy or unreasonably difficult, goals that keep changing, or goals that we don't believe in (because they were set by someone else) do not contribute much to our development through life.

For goals to succeed, they need to be shaped by our desire. We have to want them according to Burchard (2017)[33]. There also needs to be clarity of exactly what it is that we want or desire. If you want to be rich, this might refer to different things to different people. For some it will refer to money (again the amounts would change according to the country in which you are and your

[33]Burchard, B. (2017). The 4 Essentials of Achievement

lifestyle), and for others, it could refer to having rich relationships where you experience joy, comfort, and friendship

Goals will also never reach fruition if we do not approach them as formal tasks, just like you would in any other project management portfolio. One of the number one reasons why freelance contractors often do not achieve a success in the long run is that they lack the dedication and discipline to aim for and reach their goals. People are so used to having a boss that they struggle to be their own boss (if that's their goal).

According to Burchard (2017), the world (or your subconscious mind) will also throw anything and everything in the way of you reaching your goals, especially if you did not consult with your subconscious mind beforehand. In using visualization, meditation, and theta programming techniques, we can get the subconscious mind on our side, and we can create goals that are embraced by everyone on your team (your desires, your subconscious and conscious minds, and your locus of control). Alone, you will fail.

Goals have to have meaning for them to be important to us, otherwise reaching them will be pointless. So, before you state quite avidly that you want to be a millionaire, stop and consider whether this is indeed something that your mind, heart, and spirit is even interested in. Perhaps your goal could be more meaningful if you state that you want to have enough to live comfortably and be happy in your daily life. In the end, it is about what has value to you and what will satisfy your inner needs.

Your Subconscious and Your Happiness

What is happiness? Like success, we often define it in terms of stereotypical thinking. So, the question should rather be, what is happiness to you? Ackerman (2019) [34]indicates that happiness is important to living a fulfilling life, and it is often the very goal of our existence. Happiness is the antithesis of stress, and there's probably no one alive who says: "I want to have a more stressful life." Ackerman

---

[34]Ackerman, C.E. (2019). Interpersonal Effectiveness: 9 Worksheets & Examples

also alludes to the fact that happiness is not something that we can go without, and it can dramatically influence how we live and perceive our lives.

The Merriam Webster dictionary defines it as "a state of well-being and contentment: joy." But who decides what is good for our well-being and what gives us joy? Many people live in terrible conditions, experience abject poverty, and live in warzones, yet they have happiness every day. Other people live in luxury, lead lives filled with the best things, are adored by millions (like movie stars), and yet they are not happy. We can see the evidence of this lack of happiness in their drug drained eyes and failed marriages. What is the difference between the two worlds? Why would some people, who have nothing, be happy while those who have "everything", lack happiness? Happiness seems to be a state of mind and not of matter. It's about how we feel and not what we have.

Your subconscious mind is a powerful driving force in deciding whether you are happy in your present circumstances or not. If happiness is a state of mind, then we have to accept that it is not a permanent condition. It comes and goes (Ackerman, 2019). We need to work hard to reach it, and the reward of feeling happiness (if even for a few moments) is a sense of well-being and positivity that can potentially change our thinking paradigms for the better.

As you are sitting there, reading this, are you happy? Most of us will pause, and then pause some more, as we try to find evidence of happiness in our lives. In some societies, it is expected that people answer immediately that they are indeed happy, but it is not as easy as just saying "I'm happy." You may be happy at this moment (perhaps you enjoyed a lovely visit with a friend) or you may have had a good work week and, therefore, you feel happy. In the long term, you may look at your life, decide that it has been more good than bad and feel confident that you are happy. However, happiness is also based upon our perspective. If you are a negative person, you will not believe that you are happy, since your observations will strive to support your internal state. If you are a positive person and use a positive mindset, you will find observations and memories to support your internal state and the conviction that has become your personality type. Famous author and educator, Stephen Covey, wrote that "[w]e see the world not as it is, but as we are." Hence, what we feel on the inside, we will find on the outside.

Perhaps this is why some people who are miserable tend to get themselves into situations where their misery gets magnified by events (that they usually see as being beyond their control). In contrast to this, people who are innately positive and look for opportunities tend to thrive and find even more causes to be happy. How then do we change our perspectives and become happier (when we already feel like crap on the inside)?

Studies by psychology researcher Sonja Lyubomirsky (as referenced in the Greater Good Magazine by Berkeley University, found that it is indeed possible to cultivate happiness. She found that our happiness is determined by three factors:

* First, our genes make up 50% of our chances at happiness, meaning that some people are genetically more predisposed to be happy, while others are inclined to suffer depressive states.

* Second, only 10% is determined by our circumstances, which means that we can't blame where

we are or what has happened to us for our unhappiness.

- The last factor is our daily actions, which accounts for a whopping 40% of our happiness. What we do every day determines whether we will be happy or not.

There are certain activities that we can engage in to increase our happiness. These are designed to make our subconscious mind aware of our happiness (sometimes our happiness goes unnoticed). By using these activities we can improve the likelihood of experiencing happiness in our lives from now on.

Narrate your life

We are so quick to tell everyone when something bad has happened to us, yet we seem to minimize the importance of good events. We say, "I was almost run off the road by that angry taxi driver," and we fixate on this single unhappy event. If we start being our life narrator, we can choose where to focus. We can then say, "I am so grateful that I was able to miss the worst traffic and have a lovely cup of tea before starting work."

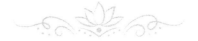

Count your blessings

Look at your life. Now decide what is in your life that makes you happy. It could be people who support you or things, like having such as a nice car. Next, imagine that all of these things and people that make you happy are removed from your life. In clinical terms, this is called mental subtraction and it teaches you to be grateful for what you have by imagining your life without it. In a Biblical sense, it is about counting your blessings. For as the adage goes, a blessing counted, is a blessing multiplied.

Build connections

Research has also found that people who are socially well-adjusted tend to be happier. They have better coping strategies and the sense of community that they share with the people in their lives gives them a sense of happiness. Our connections to other people allows us to have a support network that carries us when we are down.

Let go

Negative people tend to hold on to grudges. They go over events and people who crossed them, feasting on the regurgitated sorrow like crows. This prevents them from seeing happiness that could be theirs. Their subconscious mind is often strongly to blame for this. If you are feeling negative (and threatened), you subconscious mind will feed you the memories and emotions to match this feeling. It will even go looking for trouble. Extremely depressed people, who end up turning to self-mutilation or self-harm for release, often do so simply because it gives them a physical explanation of the pain that they feel inside. It is possible to hold a grudge against yourself. Letting go of grudges (against others and yourself) has been proven in research studies to rebuild connections and promote feelings of well-being.

Having satisfying social relationships (as well as a good relationship with yourself) has been proven to improve your happiness and develop your skills to achieve happiness as a result of your conscious actions. In other words, you can choose happiness. That choice can be made using the power of affirmations (said in repetition and most effective during theta brain wave activities). You may even wish to think of it as a form of prayer since you are asking for the changes that you desire in your life. You can take it on faith that these affirmations will work, and with your belief, they certainly will. Find a quiet spot to sit. Use a distraction such as drawing abstract lines, meditation, or even do it during a massage session (called body meditation by some) and voice these affirmations within your mind. If you are alone, you can say them aloud, as the sound of your voice (if it is firm and filled with belief) will further encourage your mind to believe these words:

"There is happiness in my day."

"I have enough; I am content."

"The people in my life fill me with joy."

"My life is filled with joy."

"Here, in this moment, I am at peace."

"I am happy."

Use these affirmations, visualization, meditation, and repetition to create the change you desire within your subconscious mind.

Your Subconscious and Your Social Relationships

Your subconscious mind has a vast and lasting impact on creating, defining, and maintaining your social relationships. Fugère (2019) finds that especially women are influenced in their romantic and sexual relationships due to their estrogen and progesterone levels. Hormones are, of course, part of the autonomic systems in the body and fall squarely within the subconscious mind's powers. Therefore, based on how our subconscious mind has regulated our hormones, we can develop a like or dislike for someone. Our reactions to someone will also be influenced by the memories we have regarding that person. To create effective and useful relationships with others, we need to learn to communicate effectively. This communication is about much more than just being well-spoken.

Communication is only effective when it is truthful and involves the other person enough to become our interpersonal communications, and this is about forming connections that mean something. Ackerman (2019) explains that communication development is not a done deal; we always keep changing and growing in effectiveness. This growth and improvement of our skills and the creation of a network of connections is made possible by the feedback we receive from the subconscious mind. It stores a myriad of recorded reactions of what is appropriate in certain situations, how you behaved in the past, and social cues and their meanings.

Being socially awkward is often as a result of having a subconscious mind that is not developed enough to guide you through the social niceties. Your subconscious mind can only give you solutions to your problems if the knowledge is there in its unlimited libraries to begin with.

Experience is, therefore, a great teacher. Today, we can even attend social classes where experts teach those who are underdeveloped in their social skills how to talk, react, touch, interact, and make conversation. Some of these are dating classes for those who are simply out of their league or have been benchwarmers their whole lives. What these classes have in common with mind programming is quite interesting. They both fill in the mental blanks. Mind programming is, however, much more effective and sophisticated. These relationship classes teach methods and habits to help people who are socially challenged to connect. Programming your subconscious mind is about breaking down the barriers that stop you from connecting, so that you are then able to form meaningful social relationships and enjoy the happiness of satisfying exchanges.

For most of us, the ultimate goal of our social interactions is to find a suitable partner, whom we can fulfill our needs with.

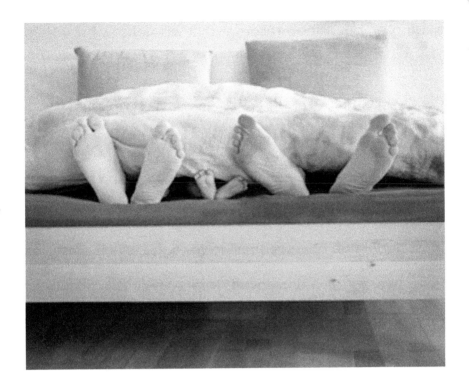

(Image 4.5)

For traditional couples, the goal is usually to procreate and continue the genetic line (this is a biological drive that our subconscious mind perpetuates). For same-sex couples, the need for acceptance, love, and validation would perhaps take precedence. However, there are many single people adopting children now (or finding other ways to have kids). In relationships, stereotypical thinking will lead to loneliness. (Image 4.5)

When applying mind programming techniques to the subconscious mind with the goal of creating better social relationships, we should use a two-fold approach. Firstly, we need to evaluate any pre-existing hang-ups that are playing on our mind's recorder that will hold us back from fulfilling our end in social relationships. Simply looking at the divorce rates across the world, as well as the prolific use of marriage counselors in relationships, tell us quite plainly that couples struggle. According to Lipton (2019), we have unsatisfying relationships because of our negative self-talk. Most people do not love themselves or believe themselves to be worthy of being loved. Hence, they are unable to express or receive love or commitment.

By using the mind programming methods that we have already discussed, it is possible to break down the mental barriers that hold back our relationship happiness. Reprogramming your subconscious mind to believe that you are worthy, that you can give and receive love, and that you deserve to be happy would be the first step. Remember the earlier quote by Stephen Covey? We see the world as we are. If we are unhappy, the world is an unhappy place. If we don't think we deserve love or relationship commitment, then we see the world as being a place without friendship or love. First, we have to change how we are, then we can begin to see the world for the possibilities that it holds.

Here's some affirmations to help you start making a social connection: (you can record these and play them back when you sleep or write them down repeatedly to "learn" them into your mind).

"I am loved, and I can love."

"My worth is mine to determine; I share my value with others."

"My life is filled with moments of joy."

"I trust in my ability to listen to others and in trusting myself."

"My partner is faithful to me, and I am faithful to them."

"My day is filled with small acts of kindness."

"I see people around me, who are a reflection of me, and I enjoy talking to them."

"People are good, like I am good, and they add value to my life."

"I can be a friend, and I have many people who are my friends."

By repeating these affirmations, you will be able to see how your subconscious mind begins to open to new possibilities, and the people that you desire to have in your life will enter it, drawn to your openness and strength.

Your Subconscious and Your Wealth

Most of us only dream of financial freedom. That elusive condition where we earn enough to live comfortably to provide for those eventualities that threaten our peace of mind. We plan to find better jobs, make investments, and even win the lottery. However, according to Assaraf (2017)[35], our monetary status is often the topic of discussion and concerns, but we never see the power that the subconscious mind offers to find or create a solution. With the problem-solving skills of the subconscious mind, we can invite wealth into our lives. It may not be as simple as winning a huge sum of money, but it can be done through dedicated efforts to change you attitudes and mindset. Putting in more time and effort at your nine-to-five job may also not be the answer. Instead, your money problems may be due to your own mindset holding you back. You can turn the tables by using affirmations to rewire

---

[35] Assaraf, J. (2017). 3 Scientifically Proven Ways To Train Your Subconscious Mind For Financial Freedom.

your subconscious mind to become more positive and, therefore, see opportunities that would otherwise be hidden from you. Often you lack the confidence and belief that there is enough wealth (money, resources, opportunities) out there to meet your needs.

Our subconscious mind can replay negative views about money, resources, and opportunities that will cloud our judgment and lead to us not seeing a way to securing the things we need. Assaraf (2017) states that "you need to slow down in order to go faster." We need to clear our minds of doubts and panic to be able to think effectively and visualize the change we desire. This can be incredibly difficult to do when you have a mortgage payment due that you don't have the means to pay. Your conscious mind will be fueled by your subconscious mind with fears of lacking enough to survive and it will be screaming that you can't do anything when you need to find a solution now! Yet, the mental clutter of our fears and negative chatter that our self-talk creates will stop us from hearing a solution.

By using mind programming techniques, you can effectively clear out the clutter and the panic and create a mental environment that will allow for your subconscious

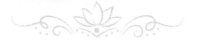

mind to begin making associations that would astound you with its ingenuity. Your imagination will begin to create a view of your life going forward that will rewire your habits. Dr. Phil is famous for coining a saying in psychology circles: "fake it 'till you feel it." This captures the essence of what you are trying to do. You need to live like you have enough, and it will happen. This doesn't mean that you go on a spending spree though! Rather, it means that you cultivate a mental attitude that there is enough, and you don't have to fight for more. You know, without any doubt, that you will be able to reach your goals (you have already seen yourself do so through your visualizations). This creates an atmosphere that some chose to call the Law of Attraction, but perhaps it is rather an atmosphere of preparedness. You have visualized yourself using opportunities to improve your wealth, so when opportunities do appear, you pursue them without hesitation or doubt, inviting success.

The process of clearing your mind BEFORE you begin to prepare your subconscious mind with affirmations, repetition, and visualization is essential. This not only triggers the all-important theta brainwaves that communicate with your subconscious but also removes the smack of "desperate" from you. As anyone in sales will tell you, a calm and confident salesman is much more effective than one who is overcome with desperation and seems to care only about making the sale. In biological concepts, it is like a herd of antelope that ostracize the wounded herd member since it attracts predators (and threats).

So, let's consider some affirmations that you can begin to introduce into your subconscious mind once you reach theta brainwaves and feel a sense of calm:

"I am strong and confident."

"I attract people, resources, and opportunities with my strength."

"All that I need for success is within my reach."

"I work hard at my goals; that hard work is being rewarded every day."

"I earn more than enough money to meet my needs."

"I have limited debts, and I have unlimited wealth."

"I am grateful for all that I have."

"I draw opportunities to me right now."

These affirmations will prepare the subconscious mind for the requests that you are making of it. It will begin to look for associations to provide you with solutions, and it will also steer the senses and autonomic reactions to make you more aware of opportunities in line with your visualizations. Your subconscious mind has the ability to remove obstacles from your path to financial freedom, and it can snap up chances that are already out there to improve your wealth. All that you need to do is to clear away the clog that you have in the machine of your mind, namely doubts and fears. Then you just have to ask (through the communication you have with your subconscious mind) and it will find ways for you to achieve all of your goals.

Conclusion

Mind programming is perhaps more in line with a revolution of the mind and you are the leader of the opposition. Your subconscious mind has tried to govern your life, and probably done a pretty bang up job of it. Now, it is time for change. The current regime based on a foundation of our past mistakes, memories, emotions, biological drives, and entrenched thinking needs to be ousted. As with any revolution, there will be those who are not in favor of the change. They will do their very best to maintain the status quo, and maintain the subconscious mind's "unthinking" leadership. These opponents are, of course, emotions such as doubt, fear, and discomfort, as well as laziness and our own inertia. Forward movement can only be achieved when we sweep clear our past concepts and bridge the habits that have lead us down paths that we didn't want. With mind programming techniques, we can begin to build new habits or information highways in our subconscious mind to recognize the opportunities and people in life that will help us reach our goals.

Where our subconscious mind was the controlling force that kept us safe from primitive fears (such as tigers) in pre-civilized times, it has been stuck doing the same job and playing the same tune (our boss has become the tiger to be feared). Today, we still believe that we are not good enough to form our own tribe (get a loving partner) or lead the hunt (find a better job), and we fear everything about the world around us that we think we can't control (without control, we are powerless and can't change).

However, with mind programming techniques such as meditation, visualization, theta brain waves, and repetition (of affirmations), we can stop that boring track from playing again. We can write our own tracks to replace track one (which was "I'm not good enough") with "I am enough and I succeed." Track two (which was "There isn't enough to go around") can be replaced with "I have enough and I make opportunities." Over time, with repetition and continued visualization, we can rewrite the script that our subconscious mind has been following and replace it with the life we've always wanted.

Make the commitment today. Commit to a reprogramming schedule of 28 days. That is the minimum length of time required to prompt neurological changes within the brain due to outside intervention (meditations, affirmations, and visualization). Identify your goals and your hang-ups, begin formulating affirmations that address your core issues, and steer your mind into the new path you've chosen. The choice to change is yours. Therefore, it works best if it is voiced in your own voice. It is the sound that the subconscious mind remembers and identifies with. Now add repetitions. Like quitting an addiction, you can't simply pay it lip service and expect results. Take your reprogramming seriously. Do it at least three times a day, with multiple repetitions to cement the new information your affirmations contain into your mind. Every time that you hear negative self-talk or emotional disturbances, it is the old regime trying to do a counter coup. Be prepared and armed with the reprogramming methods so you can end the conflict and use your subconscious mind to triumph in your life.

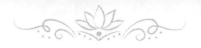

175